I0473723

The National Cancer Institute Clinical Trials Education Series

Cancer Clinical Trials Books

Cancer Clinical Trials: The Basic Workbook

The self-modulated workbook, with its accompanying activities, will help readers understand why cancer clinical trials are important, how they work, how participant safety is protected, as well as some of the reasons so few adults participate in these trials. It is designed for individuals who want to develop a basic understanding of clinical trials.

Cancer Clinical Trials: The In-Depth Program

The textbook expands on the subjects outlined in The Basic Workbook. It features additional information on clinical trials design, resources for physician participation, and referral of individuals to studies. It is designed for health care professionals and others who seek a more in-depth understanding of clinical trials.

Cancer Clinical Trials: A Resource Guide for Outreach, Education, and Advocacy

The interactive workbook provides direction and guidance for individuals and organizations interested in developing clinical trial outreach and education activities. This guide can also be used along with either/both of the texts listed above.

Trainer's Guide for Cancer Education

A manual for planning and conducting educational sessions on cancer-related topics, including clinical trials.

Cancer Clinical Trials Resources

The following resources will help support cancer clinical trials education and outreach efforts.

Publications

Low literacy **brochures** on cancer clinical trials for potential participants:

- *If You Have Cancer...What You Should Know About Clinical Trials**
- *If You Have Cancer and Have Medicare... You Should Know About Clinical Trials*

Clinical trial participant **booklets**:

- *Taking Part in Clinical Trials: What Cancer Patients Need to Know**
- *Taking Part in Clinical Trials: Cancer Prevention Studies–What Participants Need to Know**

*Also available in Spanish

Videos

- A clinical trial awareness video and speaker's guide, "Cancer Trials...Because Lives Depend on It"
- A video and discussion guide on deciding to take part in a clinical trial, "Cancer Clinical Trials: An Introduction for Patients and Their Families"

Slide Program

Three slide programs are available in PowerPoint on CD-ROM and on the *www.cancer.gov* Web site:

Cancer Clinical Trials: The Basics
Provides background on why cancer clinical trials are important, how they work, and how participants' safety is protected.

Cancer Clinical Trials: The Way We Make Progress Against Cancer
A brief community awareness presentation.

Cancer Clinical Trials: In-Depth Information
Expands on the subjects outlined above, featuring additional information on clinical trial design with resources for physician participation and referral of individuals to studies.

Ordering Information

To order these publications, contact the Cancer Information Service at 1-800-4-CANCER or log onto *www.cancer.gov/publications*. Most materials are available as PDF files on the Web site.

The Cancer Information Service
NCI's Cancer Information Service (CIS), with regional offices throughout the United States, may work with organizations and professionals to plan, implement, and evaluate culturally appropriate clinical trials education programs using the Clinical Trials Education Series. Contact the CIS at 1-800-4-CANCER.

Table of Contents

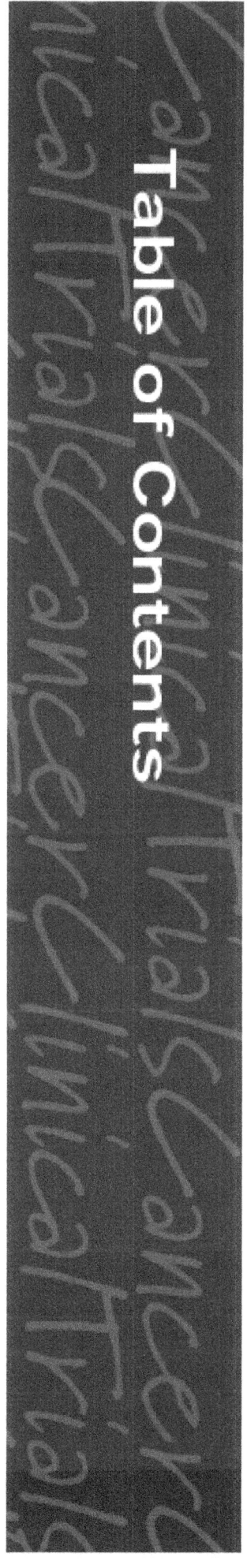

Preface

Scientific discoveries are providing more and more insights into the causes of cancer. Many of these successes are limited to the laboratory and have yet to be translated into improved care for people with cancer.

Clinical trials are a critical part of the research process. Clinical trials help to move basic scientific research from the laboratory into treatments for people. By evaluating the results of these trials, we can find better treatments and ways to prevent, detect, and treat cancer. But very few adults with cancer—only 3 percent—participate in clinical trials. We need to test the best cancer prevention, detection, and treatment ideas in the shortest time possible, and this can only happen if more people participate in clinical trials.

We know that most people understand very little about clinical trials. National Cancer Institute (NCI) research has shown that the general public is either unaware of clinical trials as a treatment/prevention option or misinformed about the clinical trial process. The reasons for this lack of understanding are complex, and there is no simple solution. We do know, however, that there are many barriers that discourage both physicians and potential participants from taking part in clinical trials.

By reading this workbook, you are already helping to overcome some of these barriers. Whether you are a cancer survivor, someone who works with people with cancer, or someone who is touched by cancer in another way—this workbook can help answer your questions about clinical trials. It will help you understand why cancer clinical trials are important, how they work, how the participants' safety is protected, and some of the reasons why more adults don't participate in trials.

With this information, you can help people in your community make informed decisions about their cancer treatment and prevention options, including the option of participating in a clinical trial.

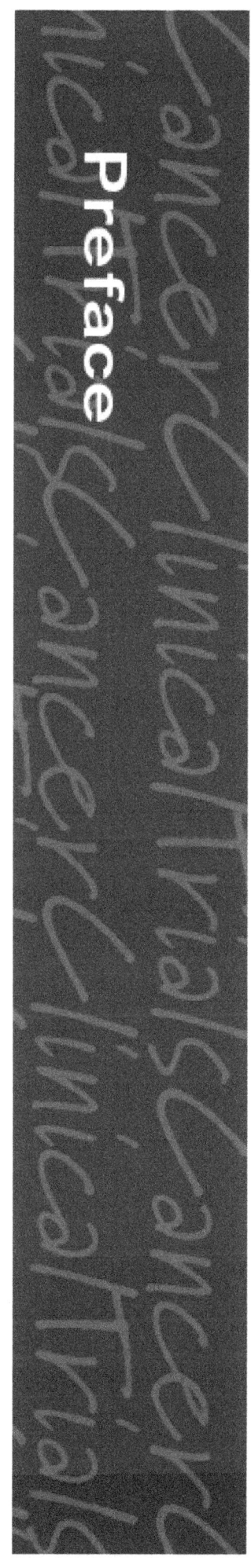

How to Use This Workbook

This workbook is designed to complement the other materials in the NCI Clinical Trials Education Series. Each section of this workbook features information about different aspects of clinical trials, usually followed by an exercise or questions. Because each section builds on the one that precedes it, it is strongly recommended that you complete each exercise to enhance your understanding of the concepts before moving on to the next section. Some of the exercises expand on concepts introduced in the text. If you are working within an organization, you may wish to read the material on your own and review the exercises with other members of your organization.

Introduction:
The Importance of Clinical Trials

Why Cancer Clinical Trials Are Important

Before reviewing how cancer clinical trials work, think about why they are important. Depending on your community, the people you work with, or the organizations you belong to, the reasons clinical trials are important to you and why more people need to participate may be different than the ones listed here.

☑ Put a checkmark next to the reasons that have the most meaning for you or write in your own reasons in the space that follows. Keep these reasons in mind as you go through this workbook.

Cancer Affects All of Us

❑ Cancer affects us all—whether we have it, care about someone who does, or worry about getting it in the future. Consider the impact of cancer in the United States[1] each year:

- About 555,550 people die of cancer—more than 1,500 people a day
- Cancer is the second leading cause of death, exceeded only by heart disease
- One out of every four deaths are caused by cancer
- About 1,284,900 new cancer cases are diagnosed

❑ Research has shown that there are many differences between who develops cancer, who dies from cancer, and who is screened and treated for cancer among men and women, and among people of different races, ethnicities, and socioeconomic backgrounds.

---

[1] American Cancer Society. (2002). *Cancer facts and figures.* Atlanta, GA.

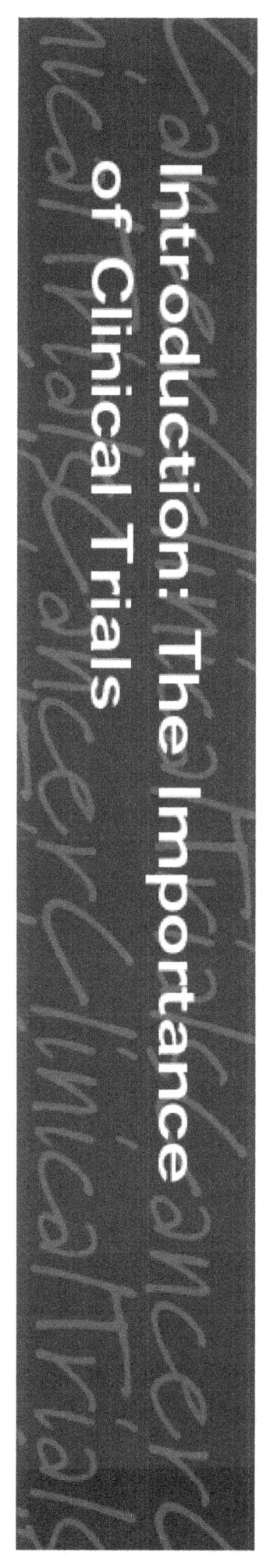

Clinical Trials Lead to Advances in Cancer Care

❏ Clinical trials are a critical part of the research process. Clinical trials translate basic scientific research results into better ways to prevent, diagnose, or treat cancer. Clinical trials are the final step in a long research process.

❏ Clinical trials contribute to knowledge of and progress against cancer. Many of today's most effective cancer treatments are based on previous study results. Because of progress made through clinical trials, many people treated for cancer are now living longer.

❏ The more people who participate in clinical trials, the faster critical research questions can be answered that will lead to better treatment and prevention options for all cancers. We will never know the true effectiveness of a cancer treatment or a way to prevent cancer unless more people are involved in clinical trials.

❏ In the past, clinical trials were sometimes seen as the last resort for patients who had no other treatment choices. This is not true; there are many clinical trials for individuals whose cancer has not spread.

Few People With Cancer Take Part in Clinical Trials

❏ Enormous improvements in treating childhood cancer have come about as the direct result of clinical trials; more than 60 percent of U.S. children with cancer participate in clinical trials. In 2000, more than 70 percent of children with cancer were alive 5 years after diagnosis, compared to only 55 percent in the mid-1970s.

❏ In contrast, only 3 percent of U.S. adults with cancer participate in clinical trials—far fewer than the number needed to answer the most pressing cancer questions quickly.

❏ According to a survey[2] in 2000, most people with cancer were either unaware or unsure that participation in clinical trials was an option for their treatment, and most of them said they would have been willing to enroll had they known it was possible.

[2] Harris Interactive. (2001). *Health Care News,* 1(3). [Poll]. Available from *http://harrisinteractive.com/about/healthnews/HI_HealthCareNews2001Vol_iss3.pdf*

Notes

1
The Clinical Trial Process

Overview

Clinical trials are research studies involving people. They seek to answer specific scientific questions to find better ways to prevent, detect, and treat diseases, and to improve care for people with diseases. Clinical trials differ by type of trial and phase of trial. Each clinical trial follows a set of strict scientific guidelines called a protocol.

Learning Objectives

By reading this section and completing the exercises, you will be able to:

- Define clinical trials
- Name the different types and phases of clinical trials
- Describe how participants are assigned to groups in "randomized" clinical trials
- Review the purpose of a clinical trial protocol and its importance
- Dispel common myths about clinical trials

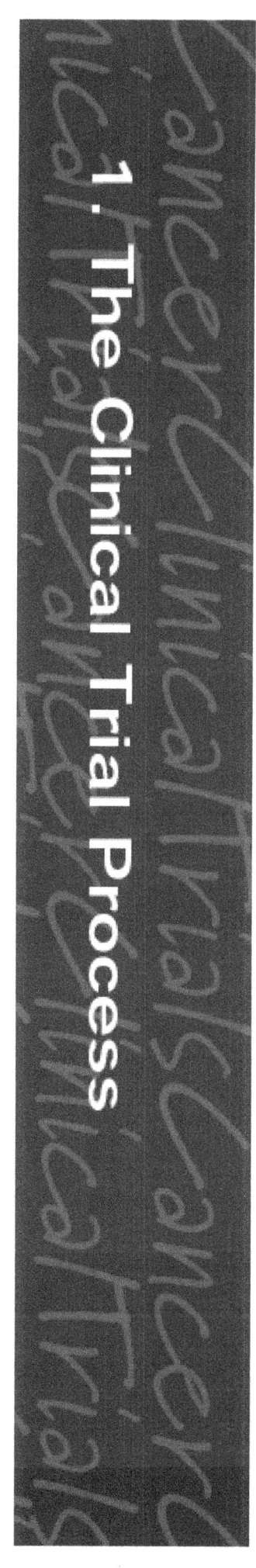

What Are Clinical Trials?

Clinical trials are research studies involving people. They are the final step in a long process that begins with preliminary laboratory research and animal testing. Clinical trials try to answer specific scientific questions to find better ways to prevent, detect, or treat diseases or to improve care for people with diseases.

In cancer research, a clinical trial is designed to show how a certain anticancer approach—for instance, a promising drug, a new surgical procedure, a new diagnostic test, or a possible way to prevent cancer—affects the people who receive it.

Cancer Clinical Trials—Types and Phases

Types of Clinical Trials

There are several different types of cancer clinical trials. This workbook will focus primarily on cancer treatment and prevention trials. Each type of trial is designed to answer different research questions:

- Treatment trials
    - What new treatment approaches can help people who have cancer?
    - What is the most effective treatment for people who have cancer?
- Prevention trials
    - What approaches can prevent a specific type of cancer from developing in people who have not previously had cancer?
- Early-detection/screening trials
    - What are new ways of finding cancer in people before they have any symptoms?

- Diagnostic trials
  - How can new tests or procedures identify cancer more accurately and at an earlier stage?
- Quality-of-life/supportive care trials
  - What kind of new approaches can improve the comfort and quality of life of people who have cancer?

Phases of Clinical Trials

Trials take place in four phases, each designed to answer different research questions.

	Phase 1	Phase 2	Phase 3	Phase 4
Number of participants	15-30 people	Less than 100 people	Generally, from 100 to thousands of people	Several hundred to several thousand people
Purpose	• To find a safe dosage • To decide how the agent should be given • To observe how the agent affects the human body	• To determine if the agent or intervention has an effect on a particular cancer • To see how the agent or intervention affects the human body	• To compare the new agent or intervention (or new use of a treatment) with the current standard	• To further evaluate the long-term safety and effectiveness of a new treatment

The trial phases are explained in the context of drug treatment trials, but the same concepts apply to most types of clinical trials.

Cancer Treatment Trials

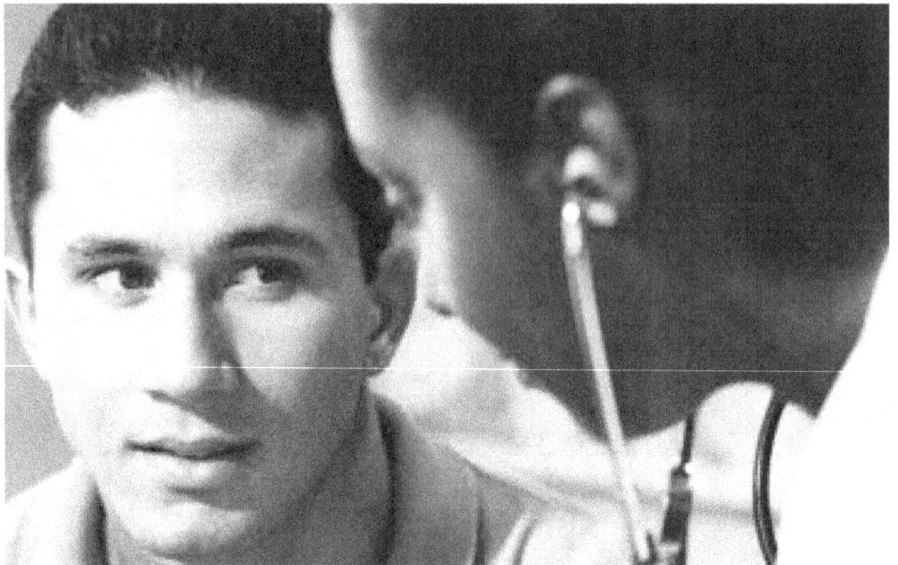

Most cancer clinical trials are treatment studies. These clinical trials involve people who have cancer. Treatment studies are designed to answer specific questions about and evaluate the effectiveness of a new treatment or a new way of using an old treatment. These trials test many types of treatments, such as new drugs, vaccines, new approaches to surgery or radiation therapy, or new combinations of treatments.

Phase 1: Looking at Safety

Once laboratory studies show that a new approach has promise, a phase 1 trial can begin. A phase 1 trial is the first step in testing a new cancer agent in humans.

An agent is a substance that produces, or that researchers believe is capable of producing, an effect that fights cancer.

In these studies, researchers look for the best way to give people the new agent (for example, by pill or by injection), how often it should be given, and what the safest dose is. These studies also include special laboratory tests such as blood tests and biopsies to evaluate how the new agent is working in the body.

In phase 1 cancer trials, small groups of people with cancer are treated with a certain dose of a new agent that has already been extensively studied in the laboratory. During the trial, the dose is usually increased group by group in order to find the highest dose that does not cause unacceptable harmful side effects, called toxicity. This process determines a safe and appropriate dose to use in a phase 2 trial. Although the primary purpose of phase 1 trials is to find the safest dose of a new agent, researchers also evaluate whether the new agent benefits people.

Toxicity refers to harmful side effects caused by the agent or intervention being tested.

Who Participates in Phase 1 Treatment Trials?

People with cancer who are eligible for phase 1 studies have no known effective treatment options, or they have already tried other treatment options. Many participate in these trials because they want to help others and contribute to cancer research. Phase 1 cancer trials usually have 15 to 30 participants.

What Are the Benefits and Risks for Phase 1 Treatment Trial Participants?

Benefits

If the new agent under study has an effect on the cancer, participants may be among the first to benefit.

Risks

Because most phase 1 trials are testing agents for the first time in humans, unpredictable side effects can occur.

Phase 2: How Well the New Treatment Works

Phase 2 trials continue to test the safety of the new agent, and begin to evaluate how well it works against a specific type of cancer. In these trials, the new agent is given to groups of people with one type of cancer or related cancers, using the dosage found to be safe in phase 1 trials.

Who Participates in Phase 2 Trials?

In general, people with cancer who take part in phase 2 trials have been treated with chemotherapy, surgery, or radiation, but the treatment has not been effective. Participation in these trials is often restricted based on the previous treatment received. Phase 2 cancer trials usually have less than 100 participants.

What Are the Benefits and Risks for Phase 2 Treatment Trial Participants?

Benefits

If the new agent under study has an effect on the cancer, participants may be among the first to benefit.

Risks
- It is important to remember that when a phase 2 trial begins, it is not yet known if the agent tested works against the specific cancer being studied.
- Unpredictable side effects can also occur in these trials.

Phase 3: Comparing a New Treatment to the Standard Treatment

Phase 3 trials focus on learning how a new treatment compares to standard, or the most widely accepted, treatment. Researchers want to learn whether the new treatment is better than, the same as, or worse than the standard treatment.

A placebo is designed to look like the medicine being tested but doesn't contain any active ingredient. Some people call a placebo a "sugar pill."

In phase 3 trials, participants have an equal chance to be assigned to one of two or more groups (also called "arms"). In a study with two groups:
- One group gets the standard treatment (control group)
- The other group gets the new treatment being tested (investigational group)

Placebos are almost never used in cancer treatment trials.

Placebos are almost never used in cancer treatment trials. In rare cases in which no standard treatment exists for a cancer, some studies compare a new treatment with a placebo.

The process of assigning participants to groups is called randomization. Additional discussion of randomization is included later in this section.

Finding Out About Standard Cancer Care

The National Cancer Institute's Web site *www.cancer.gov* contains the latest information about standard cancer treatment, screening, prevention, genetics, supportive care, and complementary and alternative medicine, as well as a registry of cancer clinical trials. Most cancer information summaries appear in two versions: a technical version for the health professional and a nontechnical version for the public. Many of the summaries are also available in Spanish.

Who Participates in Phase 3 Trials?

Participants in phase 3 studies range from people newly diagnosed with cancer to people with extensive disease. Phase 3 studies are designed to answer research questions across the disease continuum. Phase 3 trials usually have hundreds to thousands of participants, in order to find out if there are true differences in the effectiveness of the treatment being tested.

What Are the Benefits and Risks for Phase 3 Treatment Trial Participants?

Benefits

- Regardless of the group a participant is assigned to, he or she will receive, at a minimum, the best standard treatment.
- If a participant is taking the new treatment and it is proven to work better than the standard treatment, he or she may be among the first to benefit.

Risks

- New treatments under study do not always turn out to be better than, or even as good as, standard treatment.
- New treatments under study may have side effects that are worse than those of standard treatment.
- Despite phase 1 and 2 testing, unexpected side effects may occur.
- Like standard treatments, new treatments may not work for every participant.
- A participant might receive standard treatment, which might be found to be less effective than the new approach.

Phase 4: Continuing Evaluation

Phase 4 trials are used to further evaluate the long-term safety and effectiveness of a treatment. Less common than phase 1, 2, and 3 trials, phase 4 trials take place after the new treatment has been approved for standard use.

Biological Therapies: Finding Out How the Immune System Works Against Cancer

Biological therapy (sometimes called immunotherapy, biotherapy, or biological response modifier therapy) uses the body's immune system, either directly or indirectly, to fight cancer or to lessen the side effects that some cancer treatments might cause.

The immune system is a complex network of cells and organs that work together to defend the body against attacks by "foreign" or "non-self" invaders. This network is one of the body's main defenses against disease. It works against disease, including cancer, in a variety of ways.

Biological therapies are designed to repair, stimulate, or enhance the immune system's responses. Many clinical trials are now testing the use of biological therapies, such as monoclonal antibodies and vaccines, to fight cancer.

Monoclonal Antibodies (MOABs)

Monoclonal antibodies are a form of biological therapy that is now being studied in the laboratory and in clinical trials. MOABs may help the body's own immune system fight cancer by locating cancer cells and either killing them or delivering cancer-killing substances to them without harming normal cells.

Cancer Vaccines

Cancer vaccines are another form of biological therapy now being studied in the laboratory and in clinical trials.

Researchers are developing vaccines that may help a person's immune system recognize cancer cells. These vaccines may help the body reject tumors and prevent cancer from recurring. In contrast to vaccines against infectious diseases, cancer vaccines are designed to be injected after the disease is diagnosed, rather than before it develops. Cancer vaccines given when the cancer is small may be able to eradicate the cancer.

Many vaccines are not used alone, but in combination with other treatments such as surgery, chemotherapy, or additional interactions that help stimulate the immune response in general.

Cancer Prevention Trials

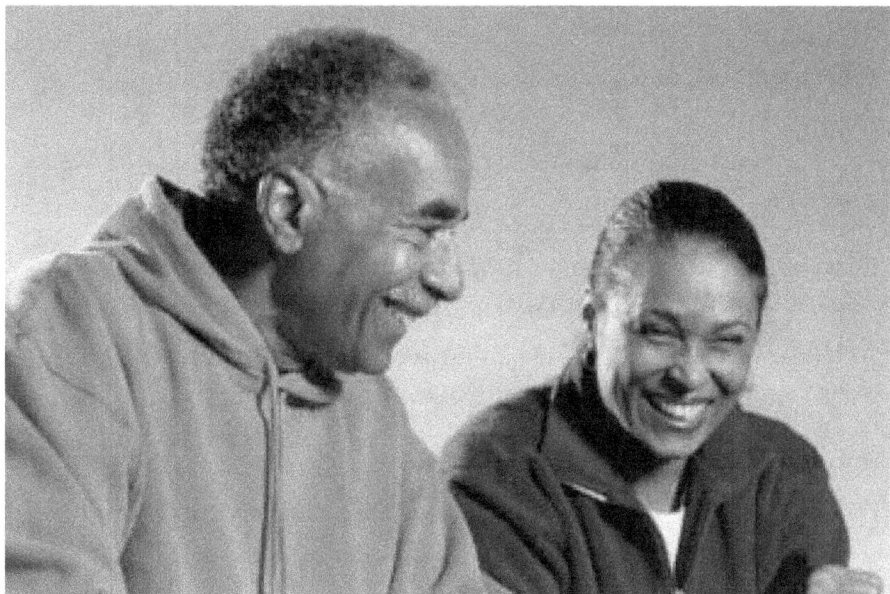

Unlike treatment trials, cancer prevention trials are studies involving healthy people who are at high risk for developing cancer. These studies try to answer specific questions about cancer risk and evaluate the effectiveness of ways to reduce cancer risk. They look at approaches to preventing cancer from developing in people who have not previously had cancer.

There are two kinds of prevention trials:
- **Action studies** ("doing something") focus on finding out whether actions people take—such as exercising more or quitting smoking—can prevent cancer.
- **Agent studies** ("taking something") focus on finding out whether taking certain medicines, vitamins, minerals, or food supplements (or a combination of them) may lower the risk of a certain type of cancer. Agent studies are also called chemoprevention studies.

Researchers who conduct these studies want to know:
- How safe it is for a person to take this agent or do this activity
- Whether the new approach prevents cancer

How Chemoprevention Trials Work

Chemoprevention trials also go through phases. In phase 3 agent studies:

- One group takes the promising new agent (called the study agent)
- The other group takes either a standard agent (already being used for cancer prevention) or a placebo

Placebos are used in prevention trials when there is not yet a known approach or standard agent for cancer prevention in the population being studied. It is important to remember that participants in prevention trials do not have cancer.

Who Participates in Prevention Trials?

Prevention trials include people who may be at risk for developing cancer. Many chemoprevention trials require that participants be at high risk for developing cancer.

What Are the Benefits and Risks for Prevention Trial Participants?

Benefits

- If the drug or intervention being studied is found to be effective, the participants may be among the first to benefit.

Risks

- New cancer prevention drugs or interventions may have unknown side effects or risks.
- The side effects of the drug or intervention may be worse and the effectiveness less than those of standard preventive measures.
- Even if a new drug or intervention is effective, it may not work for every participant.

Other Types of Cancer Clinical Trials

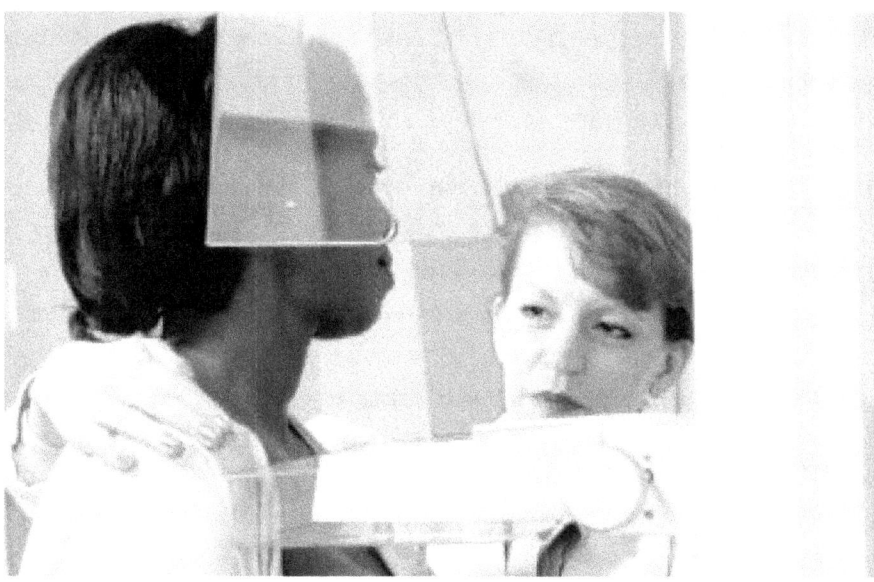

Early Detection/Screening Trials

The goal of early detection/screening trials is to discover methods for finding cancer as early as possible. For many types of cancer, detecting and treating the disease at an early stage can result in an improved outcome—a better chance to shrink the tumor, minimize its effects, or cause it to go away completely.

Ways to find cancer include:

- **Imaging tests**—tests that make pictures of areas inside the body. Imaging can be used to see if a person has any suspicious areas or abnormalities that might be cancerous
- **Laboratory tests or physical exams**—tests that check blood, urine, and other body fluids and tissues
- **Genetic tests**—tests that look for inherited genetic markers linked to some types of cancer

Diagnostic Trials

These trials focus on how new tests or procedures can better identify whether people have cancer. Diagnostic tests or procedures are done to find out whether cancer is present and, if so, where it is located in the body, if it has spread, and how much cancer there is.

Some diagnostic trials compare two or more techniques to diagnose cancer, find out how accurate they are, and see whether they can provide any new and valuable information about someone's cancer. Genetic tests are being evaluated as diagnostic tools to further classify cancers, which may help direct therapies or improve treatments for people with specific genetic changes.

Quality-of-Life/Supportive Care Trials

These trials evaluate improvements in the comfort of and quality of life for people who have cancer. They find ways to help people who are having nutrition problems, infection, nausea and vomiting, sleep disorders, depression, or other effects from cancer or its treatment. Some supportive care trials focus on families and caregivers to help them cope with both their own needs and those of the person with cancer.

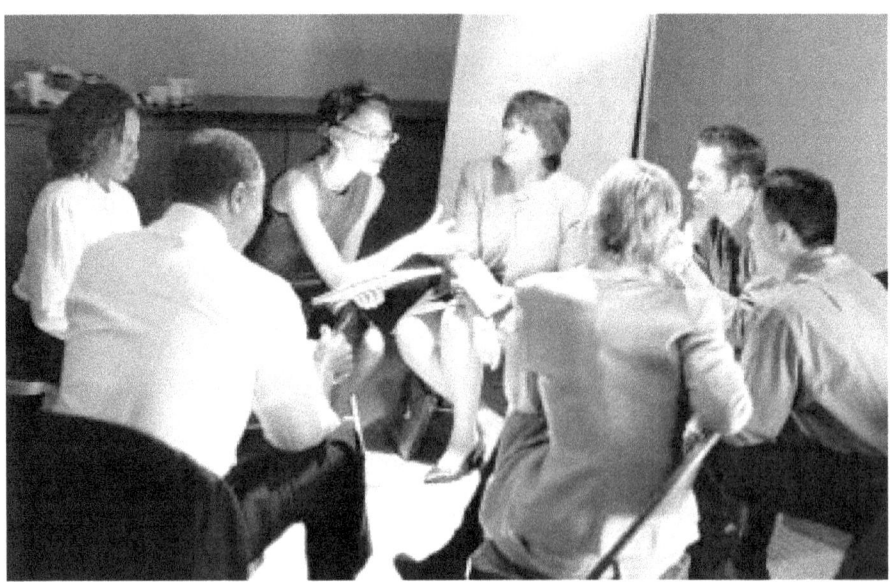

Genetics Research

Genetics studies may be a part of any cancer clinical trial and focus on understanding how someone's genetic makeup can assist in the early detection, diagnosis, or treatment of cancer. Genetic research is also being used to help develop future cancer treatments.

Population and family-based genetic research studies differ from the traditional cancer clinical trials. In these studies, researchers look at tissue or blood samples, either from families or large numbers of people, to find genetic changes that are associated with cancer. These people may or may not have cancer. The goal of these studies is to help understand what causes cancer.

Genetics research is an important part of cancer research because it contributes to the knowledge of the causes of cancer and can lead to developing new clinical trials that focus on cancer prevention, detection, and treatment.

How Participants Are Assigned in Randomized Trials

Phase 3 studies are randomized clinical trials. Some phase 2 trials may also be randomized.

Randomization is a method used to prevent bias in research. In phase 3 studies (and some phase 2 studies), participants are assigned to either the investigational group or the control group by chance, via a computer program, or with a table of random numbers. Randomization ensures that unknown factors do not influence the trial results.

Bias can be human choices, beliefs, or any other factors besides those being studied which can affect a clinical trial's results.

- The control group is made up of people who will get the most widely accepted treatment (standard treatment) for their cancer.
- The investigational group is made up of people who will get the new agent or intervention being tested.

Anyone who is considering participation in a randomized clinical trial needs to understand that she or he has an equal chance to be assigned to one of the groups. The doctor does not choose the group for the participant.

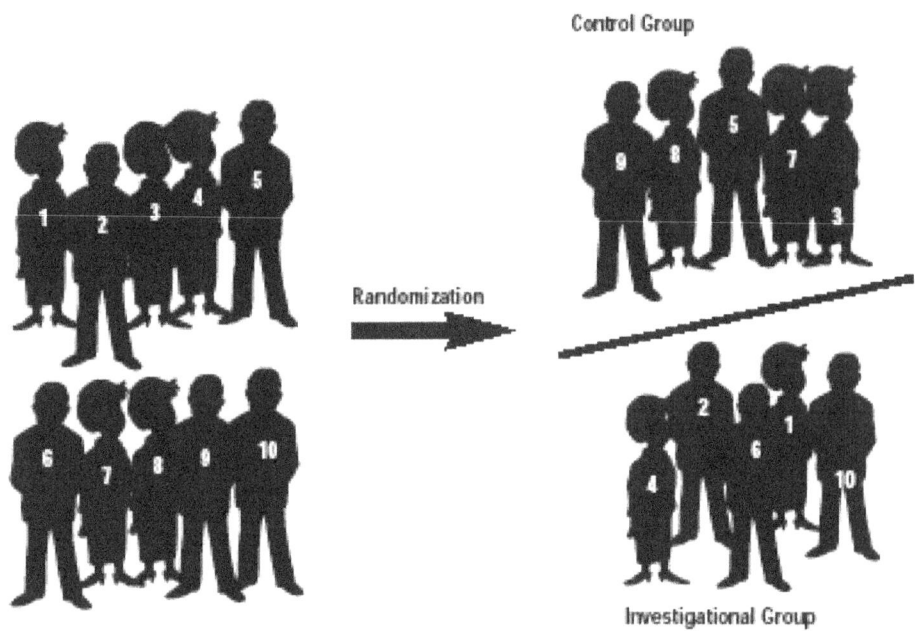

Randomization is a method used to prevent bias in research. A computer or a table of random numbers generates treatment assignments, and participants have an equal chance to be assigned to one of two or more groups (e.g., the control group or the investigational group).

Why Is Randomization Important?

If participants or doctors choose a particular group based on what they think is best, then one of the groups would likely be very different than the other, making comparison between the groups difficult. Randomization eliminates this bias because participants have an equal chance of being assigned to either group and the subgroups are as similar as possible. Comparing similar groups of people taking different treatments for the same type of cancer is a way to ensure that the study results are caused by the treatments rather than by chance or other factors.

The Clinical Trial Protocol

Clinical trials follow strict scientific guidelines. These guidelines clearly state the study's design and who will be able to participate in the study. Every trial has a person in charge, usually a doctor, who is called the principal investigator. The principal investigator prepares a plan for the study, called a protocol, which acts like a "recipe" for conducting a clinical trial.

The protocol explains what the trial will do, how the study will be carried out, and why each part of the study is necessary. It includes information on:
- The reason for doing the study
- How many people will be in the study
- Who is eligible to participate in the study (requirements might involve type of cancer, general health, age)
- Any agents participants will take, the dosage, and how often
- What medical tests participants will have and how often
- What information will be gathered about the participants
- The endpoints of the study

Endpoints

An endpoint is what researchers will measure to evaluate the results of a new treatment being tested in a clinical trial. Research teams establish the endpoints of a trial before it begins.

It is important to note that endpoints differ, depending on the type and phase of the clinical trial. Examples of endpoints are:
- **Toxicity**—what are the harmful effects of the agent?
- **Tumor response**—how does the cancer respond to the treatment?
- **Survival**—how long does the person live?
- **Quality of life**—how does the treatment affect a person's overall enjoyment of life and sense of well being?

Every doctor or research center that takes part in the trial uses the same protocol. This ensures that participants are treated identically no matter where they are receiving treatment so the information from all the participating sites can be combined and compared.

Although some people may choose to read the entire protocol before they choose to participate, the law requires that, at a minimum, participants learn about the study protocol through a process called informed consent. This information helps individuals decide whether to participate.

Guidelines on Who Can Join a Trial

Depending on the research questions, each clinical trial protocol clearly states the type of person who can or cannot participate in the trial. The reason for these guidelines includes ensuring:

- **Participant safety**—some people have other health problems that could be made worse by the treatments in a study. All potential participants interested in a trial receive medical tests to be sure that no one with special risks joins the study.
- **Accurate and meaningful study results**—some clinical trials will not take participants who already have had another kind of treatment for the cancer. Otherwise, doctors could not be sure whether the participant's results were due to the treatment being studied; the earlier treatment might have made a difference.

Other common qualifications for entering a trial include:

- Having a certain type or stage of cancer
- Having been previously treated with a certain kind of therapy
- Being in a certain age group

These criteria help ensure that trial participants are as similar as possible so doctors are confident that the results are due to the agent or intervention being studied and not other factors.

Exercises

The exercises in this workbook are optional. They are provided as tools to review the information presented in each chapter.

Exercise 1.1

Dispelling Myths About How Clinical Trials Work

Apply what you've learned about clinical trials to respond to the following myths.

A. Cancer treatment clinical trials are the treatment of last resort.

_____

_____

_____

_____

B. Only people who have cancer are eligible to participate in a cancer clinical trial.

_____

_____

_____

_____

C. Many people who join cancer treatment clinical trials get a sugar pill (placebo) instead of being treated.

_____

_____

_____

_____

D. By restricting who can go on trials, investigators keep people from getting a new treatment that could save their lives.

_____

_____

_____

_____

Answers to Exercise 1.1

A. Cancer treatment clinical trials are the treatment of last resort.

Clinical trials are not only for those with the most advanced disease. Phase 3 treatment trials, for example, can include people who have all stages of disease, from the most advanced to people newly diagnosed who have very limited disease.

B. Only people who have cancer are eligible to participate in a cancer clinical trial.

Three types of cancer trials are open to people without cancer:
- Prevention trials study ways to prevent cancer in people.
- Early detection/screening trials look at ways to detect cancer as early as possible.
- Diagnostic trials focus on ways to test for or better identify cancer.

C. Many people who join cancer treatment clinical trials get a sugar pill (placebo) instead of being treated.

Placebos are rarely used in cancer treatment trials. No one is ever given a placebo when an effective treatment is available. However, in rare cases, a placebo may be used when testing a new drug if there is no known effective treatment.

D. By restricting who can go on trials, investigators keep people from getting a new treatment that could save their lives.

There are important reasons that clinical trials have eligibility criteria:
- To protect the participant's safety. Some people have other health problems that could be made worse by the treatments in a study.
- To ensure study results are accurate and meaningful. The trial participants need to be as similar as possible so that doctors can be sure of the reasons for the results. For example, if a

participant already had another kind of treatment, the patient's response may reflect the earlier treatment rather than the one being studied.

Remember, no one knows whether the treatment being tested in a clinical trial will turn out to be better than the approaches currently being used.

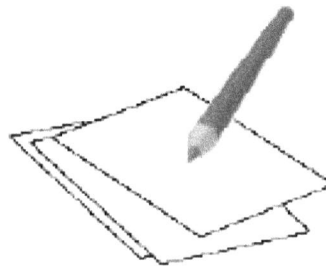

Exercise 1.2

Looking at a Clinical Trial Protocol

Apply what you've learned about clinical trials to an actual clinical trial protocol.

The following is an example of an abbreviated "patient version" protocol taken from PDQ® (physician data query), a clinical trial database sponsored by the National Cancer Institute. A "health professional" version is also available for every trial.

Please note that this trial protocol is used for illustrative purposes only; it may no longer be open to participants at the time you are reading this guide.

Although some clinical trial participants may choose to read the entire protocol before they choose to participate, the law requires that participants learn about the study protocol through a process called informed consent. This information helps them decide whether to participate.

Directions

Read the following protocol and answer these questions:

A. What type of trial is this?

B. What phase trial is this?

C. Is it randomized?

D. If someone meets the eligibility requirements, what kind of person might be interested in participating?

E. What might be of concern for someone considering participation in this trial?

Note that the protocol contains some blanks to indicate words omitted for the purpose of this exercise.

Protocol ID: NSABP-B-31

Phase _____, _____Study of Doxorubicin and
Cyclophosphamide Followed by Paclitaxel With or Without
Trastuzumab (Herceptin) in Women With Node Positive
Breast Cancer That Overexpresses HER2 (Summary Last
Modified 09/2000)

Patient Abstract

Rationale: Drugs used in chemotherapy use different ways
to stop tumor cells from dividing so they stop growing
or die. **Monoclonal antibodies** such as trastuzumab can
locate tumor cells and either kill them or deliver
tumor-killing substances to them without harming normal
cells.

It is not yet known whether combination chemotherapy
plus trastuzumab is more effective than combination
chemotherapy alone for treating breast cancer.

Purpose: _____ phase _____ trial to compare the
effectiveness of combination chemotherapy with or
without trastuzumab in treating women who have stage I,
stage II, or stage IIIA breast cancer that has spread to
lymph nodes in the armpit.

Eligibility:
• No more than 9 weeks since diagnosis
• Previous surgery to remove the tumor and lymph nodes
  in the armpit
• No previous biological therapy, chemotherapy, hormone
  therapy, or radiation therapy for breast cancer

Treatment: Patients will be randomly assigned to one of
two groups. Patients in group one will receive **infusions**
of **doxorubicin** and **cyclophosphamide** every 3 weeks for
four courses. About 3 weeks after the last course, these
patients will receive an infusion of paclitaxel every 3
weeks for four courses.

Patients in group two will receive chemotherapy as in
group one. They will also receive an infusion of
trastuzumab on day 1 of the first course of paclitaxel.
They will continue to receive an infusion of trastuzumab
once a week for 51 weeks. Some patients will receive
tamoxifen by mouth once a day for 5 years. Some patients
may receive radiation therapy daily for 5-6 weeks. All
patients will receive follow-up evaluations every 6
months for 5 years and once a year thereafter.

Key Protocol Terms

chemotherapy: Treatment with anticancer drugs.

monoclonal antibodies: Laboratory-produced substances that can locate and bind to cancer cells wherever they are in the body.

doxorubicin: An anticancer drug that belongs to the family of drugs called antitumor antibiotics. It is an anthracycline.

cyclophosphamide: An anticancer drug that belongs to the family of drugs called alkylating agents.

infusion: A method of putting fluids, including drugs, into the bloodstream. Also called intravenous infusion.

tamoxifen: An anticancer drug that belongs to the family of drugs called antiestrogens. Tamoxifen blocks the effects of the hormone estrogen in the body. It is used to prevent or delay the return of breast cancer or to control its spread.

Answers to Exercise 1.2

A. What type of trial is this?

Treatment trial

B. What phase trial is this?

It is a phase 3 trial because the description says it is not yet known whether combination chemotherapy plus trastuzumab is more effective than combination chemotherapy alone for treating breast cancer. The combination chemotherapy is considered standard treatment.

C. Is it randomized?

Yes. It says patients will be randomly assigned to one of two groups.

D. If someone meets the eligibility requirements, what kind of person might be interested in participating?

Someone who:
- Is willing to attend many chemotherapy treatment sessions
- Understands that she has an equal chance of being assigned to either group
- Is willing to be followed for several years
- Is interested in contributing to scientific knowledge

E. What might be of concern for someone considering participating in this trial?

- People will not be able to select the group they would like to participate in
- Participants must agree to be followed for several years
- People will want to know how the protocol determines who will need to:
  – Take tamoxifen daily
  – Have daily radiation treatments

2
Advancing Cancer Care Through Clinical Trials

Overview

Once a new drug or intervention is proven safe and effective in a clinical trial, it may become the new standard of practice. Everything we can tell people with cancer today about their treatment options is based on the results of clinical trials. Members of the interested public can help speed up the research process.

Learning Objectives
By reading this section and completing the exercises, you will be able to:
- Explain the process of evaluation of clinical trial results
- Describe the steps by which the U.S. Food and Drug Administration (FDA) approves a new drug
- Name some examples of clinical trials that have led to advances in cancer prevention, detection, and treatment
- Explain how members of the public can help speed up the research process

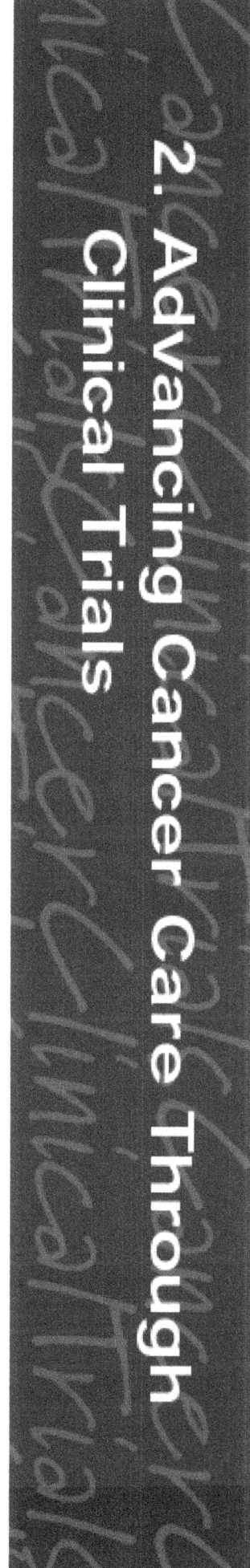

Evaluating Clinical Trial Results

After a clinical trial is completed, researchers look carefully at the collected data before making decisions about further testing and what their findings mean.

After a phase 1 trial is completed, researchers decide whether:
- There are enough data to support further study with a phase 2 trial
- Further research will be discontinued because the agent was not safe

After a phase 2 trial is completed, researchers decide whether:
- There are enough data to support further study with a phase 3 trial
- Further research will be discontinued because the agent was not safe or effective

After a phase 3 trial is completed, the researchers must look at the data and decide whether the results have medical importance. When the analysis is complete, the researchers will inform the medical community and the public of the trial results.

Peer review is a process by which experts critique a study's report before it is published to make sure that the analysis and conclusions are sound.

In most cases, a trial's results are first reported in peer-reviewed scientific journals. But if a trial's results have significant medical importance, a public announcement may be made while the formal report is being submitted to ensure that people can quickly benefit from the new advance. Particularly important results are likely to be featured by the media and widely discussed at scientific meetings and by advocacy groups.

Once a new drug or technique is proven safe and effective in a clinical trial, it may become the new standard of practice for physicians.

Approving New Drugs

By law, the Food and Drug Administration (FDA), an agency of the U.S. Department of Health and Human Services (HHS), must review all test results for new agents to ensure that products are safe and effective for specific uses.

Once a new agent proves promising in the laboratory, the drug company or research sponsor, such as NCI, must apply for FDA approval through an Investigational New Drug (IND) application. Once FDA gives approval to the sponsor, clinical trials may begin.

Once a trial sponsor feels there are adequate data from the results of the trial to support a certain use for a drug, the sponsor submits a New Drug Application (NDA) or a Biologics License Application (BLA) to FDA.

The Drug Development and Approval Process

	Preclinical Testing		Clinical Trials			Post-Clinical Trials		Total Years for Drug Approval
	Step 1 Laboratory/ Preclinical Testing	*Step 2* File IND[1] application with FDA[2]	*Step 3* Phase 1	*Step 4* Phase 2	*Step 5* Phase 3	*Step 6* File NDA[3] or BLA[4] with FDA	*Step 7* FDA Approval	
Purpose	Assess safety and biological activity in the laboratory and in animal models	Obtain FDA approval to begin clinical testing in humans after promising results in laboratory	Determine what dosage is safe, how treatment should be given	Evaluate effective-ness, looks for side effects	Determine whether the new treatment (or new use of a treatment) is a better alternative to current standard	Inform the FDA of Phase 3 data which supports drug safety and better performance over standard treatment	Review process/ approval	
All anticancer drugs (average number of years)	4.4 years		8.6 years				1.4 years	14.4 years
All drugs[*] (average number of years)	3.8 years		10.4 years				1.5 years	15.7 years

[1]IND = Investigational New Drug [2]FDA = Food and Drug Administration
[3]NDA = New Drug Application [4]BLA= Biologics License Application

[*] Classified as "new chemical entities," which exclude diagnostic agents, vaccines, and other biological compounds.
   Sources: DiMasi, J.A. (2001). New drug development in the United States 1963-1999. *Clinical Pharmacology and Therapeutics* May; 69(5); Tufts Center for the Study of Drugs Development, Tufts University; adapted from Pharmaceutical Research and Manufacturers of America.

How FDA Makes Decisions

FDA uses independent advisory committees of professionals and consumers from outside the agency for expert advice and guidance in making decisions about drug approval. By law these committees include both a patient representative and a consumer representative.

As FDA looks at all the data submitted and the results of its own review, it addresses two key questions:

1. Do the results of well-controlled studies provide substantial evidence of effectiveness?
2. Do the results show the product is safe under the proposed conditions for use? (In this context, "safe" means that potential benefits have been determined to outweigh any risks.)

For an overview of the drug approval process from start to finish, see FDA's book *From Test Tube to Patient: New Drug Development in the United States*. This book tells the story of new drug development in the United States and highlights the consumer protection role of FDA. Call 1-888-INFO-FDA or log on to *http://www.fda.gov*.

How Can the Public Influence the Drug Development Process?

As shown on the chart on page 34, it takes 15 years, on average, for an experimental drug to travel from the laboratory to U.S. consumers. Often the longest part of the process is finding people to participate in each trial phase. With increased public awareness about clinical trials, more people may be willing to participate, and more professionals may refer people into appropriate trials. This awareness ultimately reduces the time it takes for researchers to enroll participants in trials and complete them—and speeds the movement of new drugs or treatments into standard care.

Advances in Care

Most of the ways we treat cancer today are based on the results of earlier clinical trials. Recent clinical trials have resulted in the following treatment benefits for people with chronic myelogenous leukemia, cervical cancer, breast cancer, and melanoma, for example.

Chronic Myelogenous Leukemia—A New Treatment Option

In 2001, FDA approved Gleevec, offering a new treatment option for many people with chronic myelogenous leukemia (CML). Until then, bone marrow transplantation in the initial chronic phase of the disease was the only known effective therapy for CML. However, this is not an option for many people and the procedure can cause serious side effects or death. Another option, treatment with the drug interferon alfa, may produce remission (a decrease in or disappearance of signs and symptoms of cancer) for many people. But, if the drug is ineffective or people stop responding to the drug, their prognosis is generally poor.

In three short-duration, early-phase clinical trials with Gleevec, researchers found higher remission rates among people with CML than they would have expected, and the people had few side effects. Gleevec was designed to target an abnormal version of a normal cellular protein present in nearly all people with CML. The abnormal protein is much more active than the normal version and is probably the cause of the disease. By blocking the abnormal protein, called BCR-ABL, Gleevec kills the leukemia cells.

Gleevec represents a new class of cancer drugs, which target the abnormal proteins that are fundamental to the cancer itself.

Cervical Cancer—Improved Survival Rates

For many years, the standard therapy for invasive cervical cancer was surgery or radiation alone. The results of five large clinical trials showed that women with invasive cervical cancer have improved rates of survival when they receive a cisplatin-containing chemotherapy regimen plus radiation therapy.

Breast Cancer

Less Extensive Surgery, Same Survival Rate

For many years, the standard therapy for all breast cancers was a modified radical mastectomy with radiation or chemotherapy. Clinical trials showed that for women with early-stage disease, long-term survival after lumpectomy with axillary lymph node dissection plus radiation therapy is similar to survival after modified radical mastectomy.

Reduced Risk for Women at High Risk

For many years, there was no clear option for women seeking to reduce their risk of breast cancer. A large study was designed to see if the drug tamoxifen could reduce the risk of developing breast cancer in women who were already at high risk for developing the disease. The study found that those women who took the drug for up to 5 years (an average of 4 years) had 49 percent fewer diagnoses of invasive breast cancer than those who took a placebo.

Melanoma—Improved Survival Rates

According to the findings of a large, randomized clinical trial, compared to low-dose interferon or no therapy, high-dose interferon alfa-2b (Intron-A) significantly prolongs disease-free survival for people at high risk for melanoma recurrence (reappearance).

Finding Clinical Trial Results

To find trial results, look up the official name of the study and search medical publication databases, such as PDQ (*www.cancer.gov*) or PubMed from the National Library of Medicine (*www.nlm.nih.gov*). If you have trouble locating the study or searching for it, the research librarian at a university or medical library may be able to help. It often takes over a year for a scientific paper to be written, submitted, reviewed, edited, and published. If an initial search turns up nothing, try again after some time has passed.

Exercise 2

How Clinical Trials Advance Cancer Care

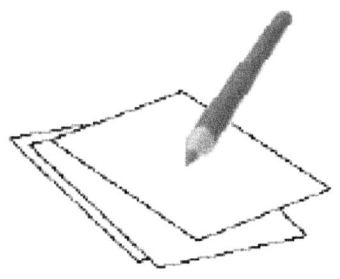

Apply what you've learned about clinical trials to respond to the following questions.

A. What happens to clinical trial results?

_____

_____

_____

B. Clinical trials answer research questions. How does this help people?

_____

_____

_____

C. Sometimes researchers decide not to continue studying an agent or to seek FDA approval. How do scientists decide when to move from one clinical trial phase to the next?

_____

_____

_____

D. How can public awareness about clinical trials influence the research process?

_____

_____

_____

Answers to Exercise 2

A. What happens to clinical trial results?

After a clinical trial is completed, researchers look carefully at the collected data before making decisions about further testing and what their findings mean.

After a phase 1 trial is completed, researchers decide whether:
- There are enough data to support further study with a phase 2 trial
- Further research will be discontinued because the agent was not safe

After a phase 2 trial is completed, researchers decide whether:
- There are enough data to support further study with a phase 3 trial
- Further research will be discontinued because the agent was not safe or effective

After a phase 3 trial is completed, the researchers must look at the data and decide whether the results have medical importance. When the analysis is complete, the researchers will inform the medical community and the public of the trial results.

In most cases, a trial's results are first reported in peer-reviewed scientific journals. But if a trial's results have significant medical importance for people with cancer, a public announcement may be made while the formal report is being submitted to ensure that people can quickly benefit from the new advance. Particularly important results are likely to be featured by the media and widely discussed at scientific meetings and by advocacy groups.

Once an intervention is proven safe and effective in a clinical trial, it may become the new standard of practice for physicians.

B. Clinical trials answer research questions. How does this help people?

Clinical trials are initiated because we don't yet know whether one treatment is better than another. Most of today's treatments for cancer are based on the results of earlier clinical trials. Clinical trials have also resulted in many new treatments and prevention options for cancer care.

C. Sometimes researchers decide not to continue studying an agent or to seek FDA approval. How do scientists decide when to move from one clinical trial phase to the next?

Clear "yes" or "no" answers are rare in science. It is particularly difficult to decide what is worth pursuing and what is not when the data are unclear. Researchers make decisions based on scientific evidence, which is why research moves in such slow and careful steps. Even if some participants in a clinical trial have a positive response to the new treatment, researchers must look at the experience of all participants when deciding whether to continue trials. For example, more people treated with the standard therapy may have better results than those treated with the experimental treatment.

D. How can public awareness about clinical trials influence the research process?

With increased public awareness about clinical trials, more people may be willing to participate. With a greater pool of participants, researchers can complete the trial more quickly and speed the development of new treatments.

E. How do clincial trials differ from unsound or alternative treatments?

Clinical trials sponsored by NCI and other reputable agencies evaluate new treatments for safety and possible benefit via IRB-approved protocols.

Complementary and alternative medicine, as defined by the National Center for Complementary and Alternative Medicine (NCCAM), is a group of diverse medical and health care systems, practices, and products that are not presently considered to be part of conventional medicine. The list of complementary and alternative medicine practices changes continually, as those therapies that are proven to be safe and effective become adopted into conventional health care and new approaches to health care emerge.

- Neither new treatments tested in clinical trials nor untested alternative treatments are known to be effective when they are initially given.
- Alternative treatements that have not been carefully studied may be harmful.
- Many CAM practices are now being evaluated within protocols for their effectiveness and safety. For more information, visit *http://nccam.nih.gov.*
- Other terms for CAM include unconventional, non-conventional, unproven, and irregular medicine or health care.

3
Participant Protection in
Clinical Trials

Overview

Many people think that participant rights are not protected in clinical trials because of past abuses of research participants. Today, Federal regulations help ensure that clinical trials are run in an ethical manner.

Participant rights and safety are protected through:
- Informed consent, a process through which potential participants learn the purpose, the risks, and the benefits of a clinical trial before deciding whether to participate. This process continues throughout the study.
- Two review panels, which approve a clinical trial protocol before it begins:
  - A scientific review panel
  - The institutional review board (IRB) that oversees clinical research at the local participating institution
- Monitoring, which continues during the trial, by:
  - IRBs, which monitor participant safety
  - Data and safety monitoring boards (DSMBs) for phase 3 trials, which perform periodic reviews of the conduct of the clinical trials and participant safety
  - Required reports to Federal agencies, which oversee the conduct of the trial

Learning Objectives
By reading this section and completing the exercise, you will be able to:
- Review key historical events regarding participant protection
- Describe how participants are protected through the informed consent process
- Explain how review boards and panels protect participants
- Demonstrate familiarity with Government regulations and agencies

History of Participant Protection

Although we now have strong safeguards for protecting those who participate in research, these protections have resulted from notorious abuses of human rights in the past. The first formal statement of protection for individuals in research emerged from the Nuremberg trials in Germany, where Nazi scientists and physicians who had conducted experiments on World War II concentration camp victims were convicted. The Nuremberg Code outlined broad concepts for the protection of human subjects and forms the basis of today's international code of ethics for the conduct of research.

In the United States, several controversial research studies highlighted the critical need for protection for those participating in clinical trials. None of these studies sought to inform the participants about the research or gain their consent.

From 1932 to 1972, the infamous Tuskegee syphilis study followed low-income African American men with syphilis but did not treat them. During the study, the men were offered free medical care and were told that they would be treated for "bad blood."

In the 1960s, two other research studies received major public attention. The first was a series of experiments with mentally retarded children; another involved debilitated elderly participants.

In response to these tragedies, regulations and policies were developed to ensure that people are told about the benefits, risks, and purpose of research for which they volunteer.

In 1976, the National Commission for the Protection of Human Subjects of Biomedical and Behavioral Research developed three basic principles governing research involving human subjects that were published in the Belmont Report. These principles, which today form the basis for human subject protection regulations in the United States are:

- **Respect for persons**—recognition of personal dignity and autonomy of individuals, and special protection of persons with diminished autonomy

- **Beneficence**—obligation to protect persons from harm by maximizing unanticipated benefits and minimizing possible risk of harm
- **Justice**—fairness in the distribution of research benefits and burdens

The Informed Consent Process

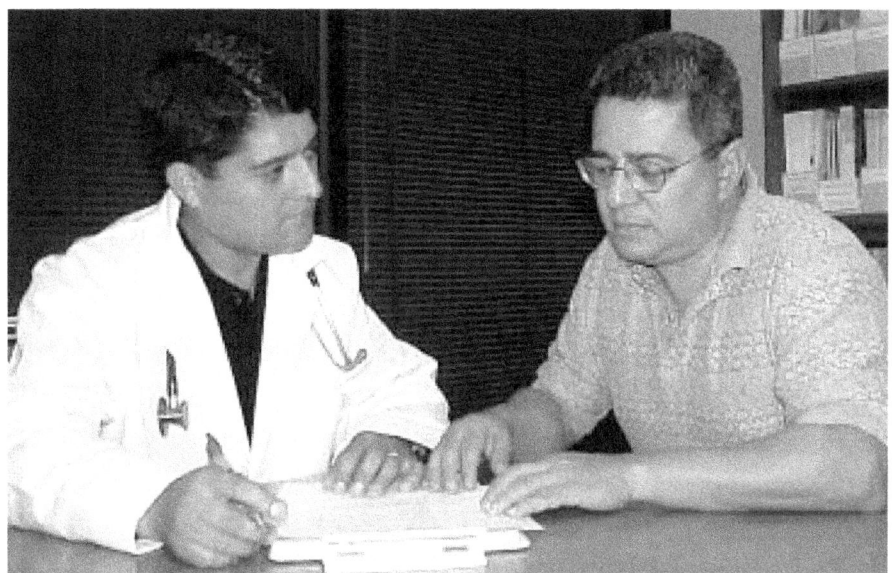

Informed consent is a critical part of ensuring participant safety in research. Informed consent is an ongoing process during which potential participants learn important information about a clinical trial. This information helps them decide whether to participate.

The research team, which is made up of doctors and nurses, first explains the trial to potential participants in understandable language. The team explains the trial's:
- Purpose
- Procedures
- Risks and benefits
- Participant rights, including the rights to:
  - Make an independent decision about participating
  - Leave the study at any time without jeopardizing future treatment

Before agreeing to take part in a trial, people have the right to:
- Learn about all their treatment options
- Learn all that is involved in the trial—including all details about treatment, tests, and possible risks and benefits
- Discuss the trial with the principal investigator and other members of the research team
- Both hear and read the information in language they can understand

Informed Consent Form

After discussing all aspects of the study with a potential participant, the team gives the person an informed consent form to read. The form includes written details about the information that was discussed and also describes the confidentiality of the participant's records. If a person agrees to take part in the study, he or she signs the form.

Although informed consent documents can vary in their length and complexity, they should all contain information on:*
- The clinical trial's nature, purpose, and duration; the procedures to be followed; and which procedures are experimental
- Reasonable, foreseeable risks and discomforts
- Benefits to the participants and to others
- Alternative procedures or treatments
- Confidentiality of records
- Procedures if the trial involves more than minimal risk (e.g., compensation, availability of medical treatment)
- Contact for questions
- Voluntary participation—that there will be no loss of benefits on withdrawal and that participants may stop participating at any time

All Government-funded trials must contain this information by law.

---

* These informed consent requirements are listed in Title 45 CFR Part 46, Subpart A.

Informed Consent Forms: Making Them Easy to Understand

The informed consent process can be effective only if potential participants understand the information given to them. In recent years, both participants and investigators have voiced concerns that informed consent documents for clinical trials were becoming too long, complicated, and difficult to understand.

NCI has issued recommendations designed to help research institutions and clinical centers write user-friendly informed consent documents. Sample templates can be found online in both English and Spanish in the clinical trials section of *www.cancer.gov.*

An Ongoing Process

The informed consent process does not end once the form is signed. If new benefits, risks, or side effects are discovered during a trial, the researchers must inform study participants. In addition, participants are encouraged to ask questions at any time about what is happening during the trial. This information helps participants make educated decisions about whether to continue participating in a clinical trial.

Pediatric Assent to Participate in Trials

Children and adolescents are not deemed capable of giving true informed consent, so they are asked for their assent to (or dissent from) participation in a clinical trial. The trial must be explained in age-appropriate language or using visual aids. Parents or guardians are asked to give informed permission for their child to participate in a trial. Assent must be obtained from all children and young people over age 7 unless:

• The child is found to be incapable of assenting

- The clinical trial offers a treatment or procedure that "holds out a prospect of direct benefit that is important to the health or well-being of the child and is available only in the context of research" (in other words, if the trial offers a treatment that is thought to be better than those currently available or if it offers the only alternative to those available).

Even in these cases, permission from the parent or guardian is required. For more information, see the clinical trials section of *www.cancer.gov.*

Weighing Decisions About Participating

People thinking about taking part in a trial should ask researchers the following questions to help with their decision-making:

- Why is this trial taking place?
- Why do the doctors who designed the trial believe that the treatment being studied may be better than the one being used now? Why may it not be any better?
- How long will I be in the trial?
- What kinds of tests and treatments are involved?
- What are the possible side effects or risks of the new treatment?
- What are the possible benefits?
- How could the trial affect my daily life?
- Will I have to travel long distances?
- Will I have to pay for any of the treatments or tests?
- Does the trial include long-term followup care?
- What are my other treatment choices, including standard treatments?
- How does the treatment I would receive in this trial compare with the other treatment choices in terms of possible outcomes, possible side effects, time involved, costs to me, and quality of my life?

Review Committees

Most clinical trials are subject to different types of review that are designed to protect all participants. Clinical trials that are sponsored by NCI—whether funded by a grant, run by a cooperative group, or run through a cancer center—are reviewed through different types of panels, including experts who review the scientific and technical merit of the proposed research. Many other clinical trial sponsors, such as pharmaceutical companies, also seek expert advice on the scientific and technical merit of their trial protocols. In addition, all federally-funded clinical trials must be reviewed by groups called institutional review boards (IRBs).

Institutional Review Boards (IRBs)

IRBs are made up of people who are qualified to evaluate new and ongoing clinical trials on the basis of scientific, legal, and ethical merit. The board members determine whether the risks involved in a trial are reasonable with respect to the potential benefits. IRBs also monitor the ongoing progress of trials from beginning to end.

Federal regulations require that each IRB be made up of at least five people; one member must be from outside the institution conducting the trial. IRBs are usually made up of a mix of medical specialists and lay members of the community, and many include members from diverse occupations and backgrounds. In most cases, IRBs are located where the trial is to take place. Many institutions that carry out clinical trials have their own IRBs.

Federal law requires IRB approval for clinical trials that are:
• Federally funded
• Evaluating a new drug, agent, or medical device subject to FDA regulation

A number of institutions require that all clinical trials, regardless of funding, be approved and reviewed by local IRBs. Potential participants considering a clinical trial should ask if it has been approved by an IRB.

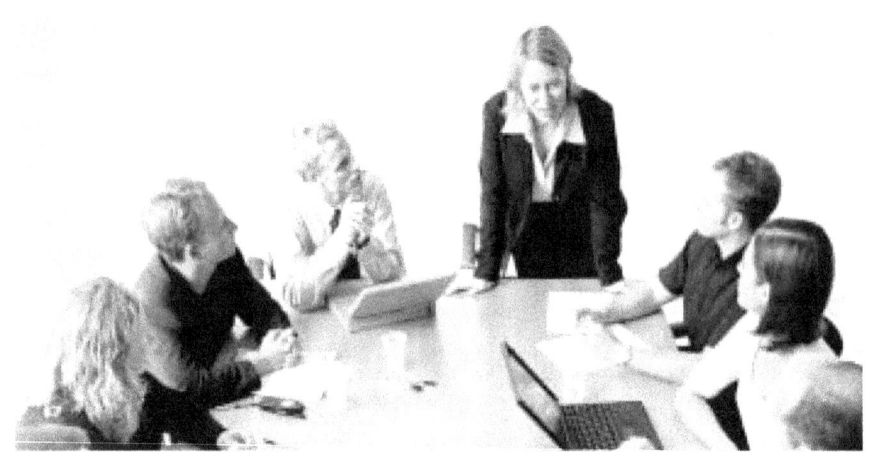

During the Trial: IRB Monitoring

If the IRB grants approval for a trial, it also must decide how frequently the trial should be reviewed once it is underway. Frequency is usually determined according to the degree of risk the trial involves.

At least once a year, the IRB must review a progress report provided by the clinical researcher in charge of the trial. The report features information about how many people are enrolled and how many have withdrawn, a description of participants' experiences, including benefits and adverse effects, and the progress to date.

Based on this information, the IRB decides whether the trial should continue as described in the original research plan, and, if not, what changes need to be made. An IRB can decide to stop a clinical trial at any time if the researcher is not following requirements or if the trial appears to be causing unexpected harm to participants.

Data and Safety Monitoring Boards (DSMBs)

For phase 3 trials, DSMBs are appointed to help ensure participants' safety. A DSMB may also be appropriate and necessary for certain phase 1 and 2 clinical trials.

The DSMB is an independent committee made up of statisticians, physicians, and other expert scientists.

The data and safety monitoring board must:
- Ensure that any risks associated with participation are minimized to the extent practical and possible
- Avoid exposing participants to excessive risk
- Ensure the integrity of data
- Stop a trial if safety concerns arise or as soon as its objectives have been met

DSMBs also monitor all trial results. If early results show clear advantages of a new drug, the sponsor of the study may choose to end the trial early and establish a protocol allowing wider use of the drug before final approval for marketing. If a drug is shown to have a strongly negative effect, the trial is stopped immediately.

In 1995, a trial of the drug tamoxifen (tamoxifen citrate) showed that the drug dramatically reduced the short-term risk of breast cancer. The DSMB and the researchers assessed the data and halted the trial so that the results could be made widely available and all women in the trial could have the opportunity to take the drug. Researchers submitted a new application to FDA, which expedited its review status. The new application was the basis for FDA approval of tamoxifen for reducing breast cancer risk.

Government Regulations and Agencies

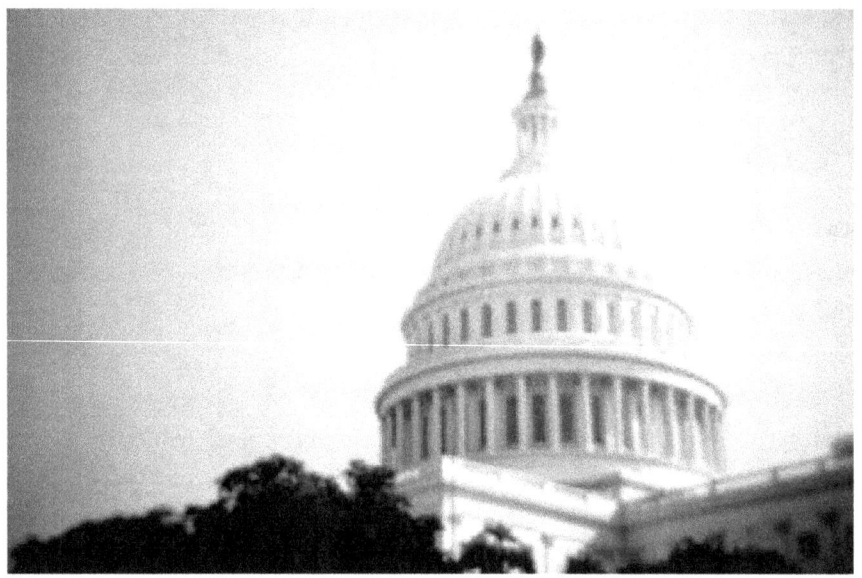

All federally sponsored trials are subject to two sets of similar regulations enforced by HHS's Office for Human Research Protections (OHRP) and the FDA to ensure the protection of people who participate. If a trial is supported by the Government and it involves an FDA-regulated drug or device, then it is subject to both sets of regulations.

People thinking about taking part in a clinical trial should ask researchers the following questions to be sure a trial is reputable:

- Who has reviewed and approved it?
- What are the credentials of its researchers and personnel?
- What information or results is it based on?
- How are the study data and participant safety being monitored?
- What happens with the results of the trial?

OHRP Regulations

OHRP protects those participating in research and provides leadership for all Federal agencies that carry out research involving people.

The OHRP enforces important regulations for participant protection in clinical trials called the Common Rule.[4] These regulations set standards regarding the:
- Informed consent process
- Formation and function of IRBs
- Involvement of prisoners, children, and other vulnerable groups in research

FDA Regulations

FDA enforces another set of regulations on participant protection in clinical trials.[5] They concern any clinical trial that involves an FDA-regulated drug or device, regardless of whether the trial receives Federal funding. FDA periodically inspects IRB records and operations to certify the adequacy of approvals, participant safeguards, and conduct of business.

Strengthening Government Oversight

Although breaches in participant protection seldom occur, recent discoveries of inadequate participant protection have taken place. Beginning in 2000, HHS began to take additional steps to:
- Strengthen regulations concerning participant safety
- Strengthen Government oversight of medical research
- Reinforce clinical researchers' responsibilities to follow Federal research guidelines

[4] Title 45 CFR Part 46, Subpart A
[5] Title 21 CFR Part 50, 56

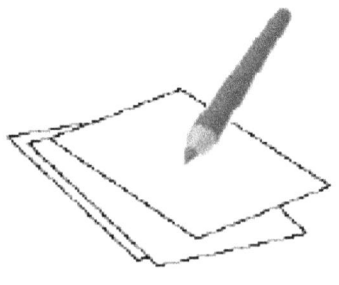

Exercise 3

Participant Protection

How would you respond to the following questions?

A. Aren't people who join clinical trials just "guinea pigs" for research without protections?

_____

_____

_____

B. Can a person be put on a clinical trial without his or her knowledge?

_____

_____

_____

C. If someone is in a phase 3 trial and it is found that there is a clear advantage for the participants in the other group, what happens?

_____

_____

_____

D. What happens if someone wants to stop participating in a trial?

_____

_____

_____

Answers to Exercise 3

A. Aren't people who join clinical trials just "guinea pigs" for research?

Many safeguards are in place for people who join cancer trials. All clinical trial participants go through the informed consent process. Informed consent is an ongoing process in which people learn important information about a clinical trial. This information helps them decide whether to participate.

The trial is also monitored by an institutional review board (IRB) and, if the study is a phase 3 clinical trial, by a data and safety monitoring board (DSMB).

In response to breaches in protection that have been recently identified and reported in the media, in 2000, the U.S. Department of Health and Human Services took additional steps to strengthen Government oversight of medical research and to reinforce clinical researchers' responsibility to follow guidelines.

B. Can a person be put in a clinical trial without his or her knowledge?

No. The researchers running the trial are required by law to present and explain the study as part of the informed consent process. This process includes:

- Signing an informed consent document (so that people know they are entering a study)
- Discussing with the research team what the trial entails
- Understanding the potential risks and benefits of participating

Although reputable researchers do not fool people or sign them up against their will, sometimes people have difficulty understanding the information they need to know about a trial before agreeing to join. For many people, it is important to ask a friend or family member to come with them to be sure that all important questions are raised. Taking notes or using a tape recorder can also help.

C. **If someone is in a phase 3 trial and it is found that there is a clear advantage for the participants in the other group, what happens?**

The DSMB would report the information to the study sponsor. If early results show that there is a clear advantage for one of the groups, the sponsor may choose to end the trial early and establish a protocol allowing wider use of the drug before final approval for marketing.

D. **What happens if someone wants to stop participating in a trial?**

Under the informed consent process, a person has the right to discontinue their participation in a trial at any time. A participant's decision to leave a clinical trial does not jeopardize future treatment, and the participant will have the chance to discuss other treatments, or care with a doctor from the trial. The person may be referred back to his or her primary doctor for standard care.

4
Barriers to Clinical Trial Participation

Overview

Many people with cancer do not participate in clinical trials. Common barriers to participating include lack of awareness; lack of access; fear, distrust, or suspicion of research; and financial and personal concerns.

Learning Objectives
By reading this section and completing the exercise, you will be able to:
- Identify some barriers people face when considering participation in clinical trials
- Describe some of the costs associated with clinical trials

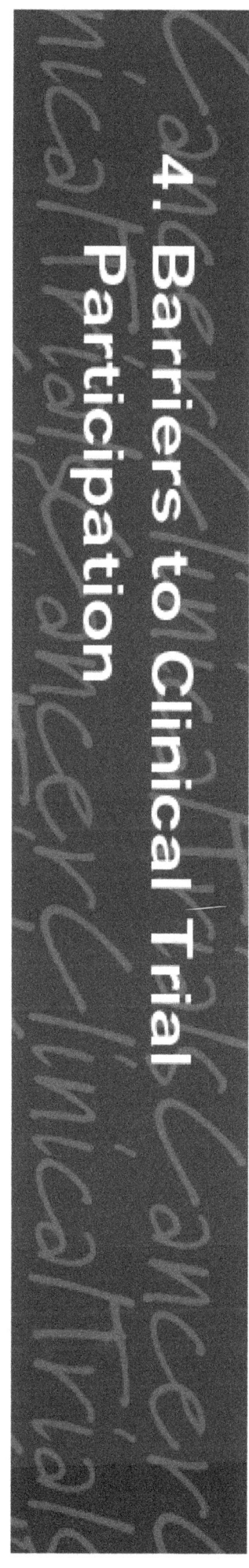

Participation in Clinical Trials

"Only 3 percent of adult cancer patients in the United States participate in clinical trials—far fewer than the number needed to answer the most pressing cancer questions quickly."*

Reflecting on the quote above, why do you think more people don't participate in clinical trials?

_____

_____

_____

_____

_____

Compare your answer to the information in this section.

* Excerpted from an American Society of Clinical Oncology news release, 1999.

Barriers for Health Care Professionals

- **Lack of awareness of appropriate clinical trials.** Physicians are not always aware of available clinical trials. Some may not be aware of the local resources, or some may assume that none would be appropriate for their patients.
- **Unwillingness to "lose control" of a person's care.** Most doctors feel that the relationship they have with their patients is very important. They want what is best for the patient, and if the person must be referred elsewhere to participate in a trial, doctors fear they may lose control of the person's care.
- **Belief that standard therapy is best.** Many health care providers may not adequately understand how clinical trials are conducted or their importance. Some believe that the treatment in clinical trials is not as good as the standard treatment. They also might be uncomfortable admitting that there is uncertainty about which treatment is best in a phase 3 clinical trial.
- **Belief that referring to and/or participating in a clinical trial adds an administrative burden.** The length and details of most research protocols may deter providers from participating in

clinical trials. The possibility of incurring additional costs and expenses that might be inadequately reimbursed is a deterrent for many.

- **Concerns about the person's care or how the person will react to the suggestion of clinical trial participation.**

Barriers for the General Population

- **Lack of awareness of clinical trials.** Research has consistently shown that most people with cancer are not aware of the option to participate in clinical trials.
- **Lack of access to trials.** The reality or the perception that there are no trials nearby deters many potential participants. In addition, seeking care at a distant trial site presents time and travel barriers.
- **Fear, distrust, or suspicions of research.** For many people, the loss of control (not choosing their treatment) that comes with entering a randomized trial is too great. Many also fear being treated like "guinea pigs" or being "experimented upon," as well as not receiving treatment for their cancer. People may have a general lack of trust in the medical profession based on past negative experiences or the knowledge of historical abuses of research participants.
- **Practical or personal obstacles.** Costs of being away from work and family may be deterrents for some people. Others may not wish to leave the care of their own physician. People from certain racial or ethnic groups or who are medically underserved may feel that care within a trial will not be sensitive to their needs. Others may feel that recruitment strategies are not sensitive to their needs. Still others may believe that standard care is better than the treatment available in a trial.
- **Insurance or cost problems.** Another deterrent is the fear of being denied insurance coverage for participation in a clinical trial. If a person is uninsured, the cost of trial participation is an issue.
- **Unwillingness to go against personal physician's wishes.**

A Survey on Clinical Trial Barriers

A survey of almost 6,000 people with cancer conducted in 2000 took a look at why so few adults participate in cancer clinical trials. Some of the highlights included:

- About 85 percent of people with cancer were either unaware or unsure that participation in clinical trials was an option, though about 75 percent of these people said they would have been willing to enroll had they known it was possible.
- Of those who were aware of the clinical trial option, most declined to participate because they believed common myths about clinical trials. They either thought that
  - The medical treatment they would receive in a clinical trial would be less effective than standard care
  - They might get a placebo
  - They would be treated like a "guinea pig"
  - Their insurance company would not cover costs
- People who received treatment through a clinical trial found it to be a very positive experience:
  - Ninety-seven percent said they were treated with dignity and respect and that the quality of care they received was "excellent" or "good"
  - Eighty-six percent said their treatment was covered by insurance

Source: Harris Interactive. (2001). *Health Care News*, 1(3). [Poll]. Available from *http://harrisinteractive.com/about/healthnews/HI_HealthCareNews2001Vol_iss3.pdf*

Supported by the Coalition of National Cancer Cooperative Groups, the Cancer Research Foundation of America, the Cancer Leadership Council, and the Oncology Nursing Society.

Barriers for Racially or Ethnically Diverse Populations

Additional barriers exist for people who are from certain ethnic/racial backgrounds or who are medically underserved. The following list is not meant to be a comprehensive overview of all barriers associated with clinical trials, and what is outlined should not be generalized to all diverse populations.

More information about these groups, as well as ideas for addressing these barriers, can be found in *Cancer Clinical Trials: A Resource Guide for Outreach, Education, and Advocacy.*

Diverse U.S. Populations: Definitions

Diverse populations include minority ethnic and racial groups designated by the U.S. Government, such as:

- American Indian or Alaska Native
- Asian American
- Black or African American
- Hispanic or Latin American
- Native Hawaiian or other Pacific Islander

Ethnically diverse populations are growing rapidly; in the 2000 Census, about 25 percent of the U.S. population reported their race as something other than White.

NCI's working definition of diverse populations also includes medically underserved populations. Medically underserved populations are those that lack easy or any access to, or don't make use of, high-quality cancer prevention, screening and early detection, treatment, or rehabilitation services. These may include people of any racial or ethnic group who live in rural areas or who have low income or literacy levels. Medically underserved groups are generally characterized as experiencing higher cancer mortality rates and insufficient participation rates in cancer control programs.

Specific Barriers

- **Long-standing fear, apprehension, and skepticism** exist among some minority populations about medical research because of abuses that have happened in the past (e.g., the legacy of the Tuskegee syphilis study). Among these populations, there is often widespread fear and distrust of the medical care system as a result of discrimination, indifference, and disrespect. Many feel that they do not want to give up rights or lose power to be "experimented on." Others may be skeptical about the quality of care that would be provided in a clinical trial. Some may find that trial recruitment strategies are not sensitive to their needs.

- **Doctors may not mention clinical trials as an option** for cancer care. As noted above, many physicians do not refer people to clinical trials. However, some physicians may avoid suggesting a clinical trial to people who belong to racial or ethnic minorities out of concern that they would seem insensitive. Moreover, some physicians may inadvertently discriminate against older people or those from certain ethnic or cultural backgrounds.

- **People from various cultural or ethnic backgrounds may hold values and beliefs that may be different than those of Western medicine.** Many people have a cultural belief that Western medicine cannot address their health concerns. Different ethnic and cultural views of health and disease (e.g., fatalism, family decisions about treatment, use of "traditional healers," prayer, herbal medicines, or use of complementary/alternative health practices) may make clinical trials a less attractive treatment option. For prevention trials, many may feel that the risk of a potential disease and its consequences may be less important than meeting daily needs.

- **Language or literacy barriers** may make it difficult for some people to understand and consider participating in clinical trials. The complexity of forms, including informed consent documents, may also be a barrier to those considering participation in a clinical trial. Translation can also be difficult if the person translating information has not had specialized training.

- **Additional access problems** confront many people. Depending on where they live or their access to transportation, people may have difficulty getting back and forth from a clinical trial site. Those with low incomes may find it difficult to take time off work or find appropriate childcare. Other barriers, such as a lack of health insurance or a source of health care, clearly present difficulties in accessing trials.

For solutions to barriers for racially and ethnically diverse populations, see NCI's *Cancer Clinical Trials: A Resource Guide for Outreach, Education, and Advocacy.*

Cost Barriers

The costs associated with clinical trials can be a barrier for many professionals and the public. Physicians are often concerned about reimbursement related to the expenses of either caring for people enrolled in trials or offering trials within their practice. Potential trial participants often fear that their insurance company will not cover their participation in a clinical trial. Those who are uninsured will need to know how their participation in a trial will be covered.

There are two types of costs associated with clinical trials—participant care costs and research costs.

Participant Care Costs

Participant care costs include:
- **Usual care costs**, such as doctor visits, hospital stays, clinical laboratory tests, and x-rays, occur whether someone is participating in a trial or receiving standard treatment.
- **Extra care costs** are those associated with clinical trial participation, such as additional tests that may be required.

These costs may or may not be covered by a participant's health plan.

Research Costs

Research costs include costs associated with conducting the trial, such as:
- Data collection and management
- Research physician and nurse time

- Analysis of results
- Clinical laboratory tests and x-rays
- Cost of the agent being tested

Most of the time, research costs are covered by the sponsoring organization or by a pharmaceutical company.

Health Plan Coverage—Treatment Trials

Health insurance companies and managed care providers do not always cover all participant care costs in a study. What they cover varies by plan and by trial. In general, the most important factor in whether a treatment is covered is a health plan's judgment as to whether the therapy is "established" or "investigational."

Health plans often claim that paying for clinical trials will be too costly. However, several studies in 1999 and 2000 found that participant care costs for clinical trials are not much higher than costs for people who are not enrolled in trials.[*]

Health Plan Coverage—Chemoprevention Trials

Although participants receive preventive agents free of charge, coverage for required medical tests is often at issue. For example, pre-entry tests are paid for by the trial at some (but not all) institutions. However, the individual may need a retest if the pre-entry test shows any suspicious findings, and the retest costs may not be covered. If a person belongs to a managed care organization, coverage for the retest will be denied if the primary care gatekeeper has not authorized it, regardless of other considerations. In addition, some trials require certain preventive screening tests annually, such as mammograms, but not all insurers cover preventive screening tests for all participants.

*Bennett, C. L., et al. (2000). Evaluating the financial impact of clinical trials in oncology: Results from a pilot study from the Association of American Cancer Institutes/ Northwestern University Clinical Trials Costs and Charges Project. *Journal of Clinical Oncology*, 18, 2805-2810. Fireman, B., et al. (2000). Cost of care for patients in cancer clinical trials. *Journal of the National Cancer Institute*, 92, 136-142. Wagner, J. L., et al. (1999). Incremental costs of enrolling cancer patients in clinical trials: A population-based study. *Journal of the National Cancer Institute*, 91, 847-853.

In considering options, interested persons should ask trial personnel what the experience to date has been in the trial they are considering. They should ask specifically about the type of insurance involved. People may even be able to get examples of how their employer or managed care plan has responded.

Potential participants should call NCI's Cancer Information Service at 1-800-4-CANCER or visit the clinical trials section of *www.cancer.gov*, which features tips and information about organizations to help with clinical trials coverage.

> People considering a trial should work with a doctor or social worker to get specific information from the facility running the trial. They should ask questions such as:
> - What parts of treatment, if any, does the trial provide free of charge?
> - What parts of treatment must be paid for by me or by my health plan?
> - What is the situation for people who have no health insurance?
> - Will my total charges be higher as a clinical trial participant than if I opt for standard care?
> - How successful are you in getting insurers to cover the patient care costs in the study I am considering?
> - Are there other resources or organizations you can recommend to help me meet the fees or to provide services such as free transportation?

Legislation and Policies

Despite interest at the Federal level, as of 2001, no legislation has been passed to require private third-party payers to uniformly cover all clinical trial costs. However, there have been several important developments at the Federal level regarding clinical trial coverage:
- Medicare reimburses for all routine participant care costs for its beneficiaries participating in clinical trials.

- Beneficiaries of TRICARE, the Department of Defense's health program, are covered for NCI-sponsored phase 2 and phase 3 prevention and treatment clinical trials.
- Department of Veterans Affairs (VA) allows eligible veterans to participate in a broad range of NCI clinical trials across the country. The agreement covers all phases and types of NCI-sponsored trials.

Many states have also passed legislation or developed policies that require health plans to cover clinical trial costs. For an updated legislation listing, see the clinical trials section of *www.cancer.gov*.

Exercise 4

Barriers to Participation

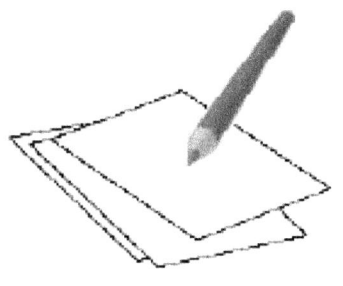

A. Do doctors discuss clinical trials as options for their patients?

_____

_____

_____

B. If a doctor cannot or will not refer a person to a clinical trial, can the person or family make the call directly?

_____

_____

_____

C. Is it more expensive to participate in a clinical trial compared to standard treatment? Are clinical trials covered by insurance?

_____

_____

_____

D. Are chemoprevention trials covered by insurance? If so, will participants compromise their coverage by entering trials for those at "high risk" for cancer?

_____

_____

_____

Answers to Exercise 4

A. Do doctors discuss clinical trials as options for their patients?

Some health professionals may not discuss clinical trials with their patients for the following reasons:
* They are not aware of clinical trials
* They are unwillingly to lose control of a person's care
* They believe that standard therapy is best
* They cannot find a trial which is compatible with the person's clinical situation

No matter what the situation, people with cancer have the right to consider all possible treatment options before deciding which treatment option is right for them.

B. If a doctor cannot or will not refer a person to a clinical trial, can the person or family make the call themselves?

Decisions about eligibility for a trial can be complicated and require very specific medical information on a person's condition. Therefore,
* It is preferable to have the contact made by a health care professional familiar with the case
* Participants calling researchers directly may not have all the information needed to make eligibility decisions
* If a physician is unwilling to make contact with clinical trial investigators, the best alternative may be to request a referral to another physician

C. Is it more expensive to participate in a clinical trial compared to standard treatment? Are clinical trials covered by insurance?

There are two kinds of costs associated with clinical trials:
* Patient care costs
  - May be covered by a person's health plan
  - Include usual care cost items like doctor visits, hospital stays, clinical laboratory tests, and x-rays, which occur whether someone is participating in a trial or receiving standard treatment.

- Research costs
  - Usually covered by the trial's sponsor
  - Include extra care costs associated with clinical trial participation such as additional tests

- Some health plans cover the costs associated with clinical trial participation; other companies will not reimburse for "experimental therapies"
- Decisions are usually made on a case-by-case basis
- Some clinical trial sponsors work with health plans to get reimbursement
- People interested in clinical trial participation should ask the trial team what their experience with reimbursement for this trial has been
- Clinical trial participants may also contact NCI's Cancer Information Service at 1-800-4-CANCER or visit the clinical trials section of *www.cancer.gov* for information on organizations that may help with clinical trial coverage

D. Are chemoprevention trials covered by insurance? If so, will participants compromise their coverage by entering trials for those at "high risk" for cancer?

There is no comprehensive data on insurance problems related to entering a chemoprevention trial, but some issues have been reported:
- Participants receive prevention agents free of charge
- Coverage for medical tests can be an issue
- Some institutions will pay for the initial tests, but not all
- If a re-test is needed it may not be covered, especially if it has not been authorized by a primary care gatekeeper
- Prevention trials may require more frequent screening exams (such as a mammogram or colonoscopy), and insurers may not want to cover a test given more frequently than their guidelines require (for example every six months versus every year)
- Many insurance companies have policies on "pre-existing conditions," so entering a trial for those at "high risk" could make it harder or more expensive to get health and life insurance in the future

- Some states have laws about pre-existing conditions and Federal law forbids companies to deny health care to people with pre-existing conditions. It remains unclear how insurers will handle "high risk" conditions.
- Participants may contact NCI's Cancer Information Service at 1-800-4-CANCER or visit the clinical trials section of *www.cancer.gov* for information on organizations that help with clinical trials coverage and insurance questions.

5
Finding Clinical Trials

Overview

Cooperative groups, cancer centers, hospitals, and local physician offices conduct clinical trials. NCI, pharmaceutical companies, and other groups may fund them. They take place in diverse locations all over the country.

When locating clinical trials, it is important to remember that no single resource, including those from NCI, lists every cancer clinical trial.

Learning Objectives
By reading this section and completing the exercises, you will be able to:
- Identify who sponsors cancer clinical trials
- Describe the role of NCI in how clinical trials are conducted at sites throughout the United States
- Describe the process by which people can be referred to clinical trials
- Explain ways to locate clinical trials

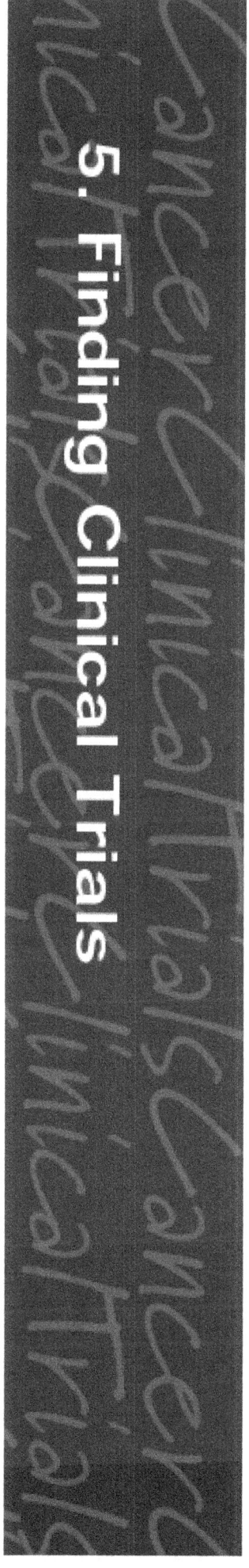

Organizations That Sponsor Clinical Trials

NCI, pharmaceutical companies, medical institutions, and other organizations sponsor clinical trials. NCI often partners with pharmaceutical companies to develop new agents.

Regardless of sponsor, clinical trials take place at universities, large medical centers, small hospitals, and doctors' offices. Individual physicians at cancer centers and other medical institutions can also sponsor clinical trials themselves.

NCI-Sponsored Clinical Trials

NCI sponsors many clinical trials around the country that are conducted through four different programs:
1. Clinical Trials Cooperative Group Program
2. Community Clinical Oncology Program (CCOP) and the Minority-Based Community Clinical Oncology Program (MBCCOP)
3. Cancer Centers Program
4. Clinical Grants Program

All NCI-sponsored trials must meet all FDA and Office for Human Research Protections (OHRP) regulations for participant protection in clinical trials.

Clinical Trials Cooperative Group Program

Clinical trials are often conducted through NCI cooperative clinical trial groups, which are networks of institutions that jointly carry out large clinical trials following the same protocols. Members of these groups include:
- University hospitals
- Cancer centers
- Community physicians and community hospitals

Cooperative groups develop and conduct new clinical trials that follow national priorities for cancer research. They conduct phase 3 trials as well as phase 2 trials.

Some of the groups are categorized by type of cancer, others by type of treatment, and at least one by age of participants. Other groups are regional or focus on several cancer types.

There are 12 groups in the Clinical Trials Cooperative Group Program:
  1. American College of Surgeons Oncology Group (ACOSOG)
  2. Cancer and Acute Leukemia Group B (CALGB)
  3. Children's Cancer Study Group (CCSG)
  4. Eastern Cooperative Oncology Group (ECOG)
  5. Gynecologic Oncology Group (GOG)
  6. Intergroup Rhabdomyosarcoma Study Group (IRSG)
  7. National Surgical Adjuvant Breast and Bowel Project (NSABP)
  8. National Wilms Tumor Study Group (NWTSG)
  9. North Central Cancer Treatment Group (NCCTG)
 10. Pediatric Oncology Group (POG)
 11. Radiation Therapy Oncology Group (RTOG)
 12. Southwest Oncology Group (SWOG)

For more information about the Cooperative Group program, see *http://ctep.info.nih.gov.*

Community Clinical Oncology Programs (CCOPs) and Minority-Based CCOPs (MBCCOPs)

These programs allow community physicians to work with scientists conducting NCI-supported clinical trials. Participation in the CCOP benefits lay people and health professionals in the community as well as scientists in research centers.

The MBCCOP provides members of ethnic and racial minorities with access to state-of-the-art cancer treatment, prevention, and control technology.

Cancer Centers Program

NCI cancer centers conduct clinical trials under an NCI-approved protocol review and surveillance mechanism.

The Cancer Centers Program consists of more than 50 NCI-designated cancer centers involved in many different cancer research efforts. Cancer centers also participate in at least one cooperative group.

Clinical Grants Program

Many clinical trial protocols are carried out under the direct support of an NCI peer-reviewed grant.

Industry-Sponsored Trials

Pharmaceutical and biotech companies conduct their own trials, both locally and nationally. They may have as partners universities, hospitals, NCI, or local doctors. These trials are subject to the companies' own review panels and to an IRB, which may be local or national in scope.

Referrals to Clinical Trials

Once someone is diagnosed with cancer, the health care provider may suggest several possible treatment options, one of which may be a clinical trial. Similarly, health care providers may offer people at high risk for cancer several options for prevention, including a clinical trial. If a person finds that his or her physician does not participate in clinical trials, the person can request a referral to a physician who does.

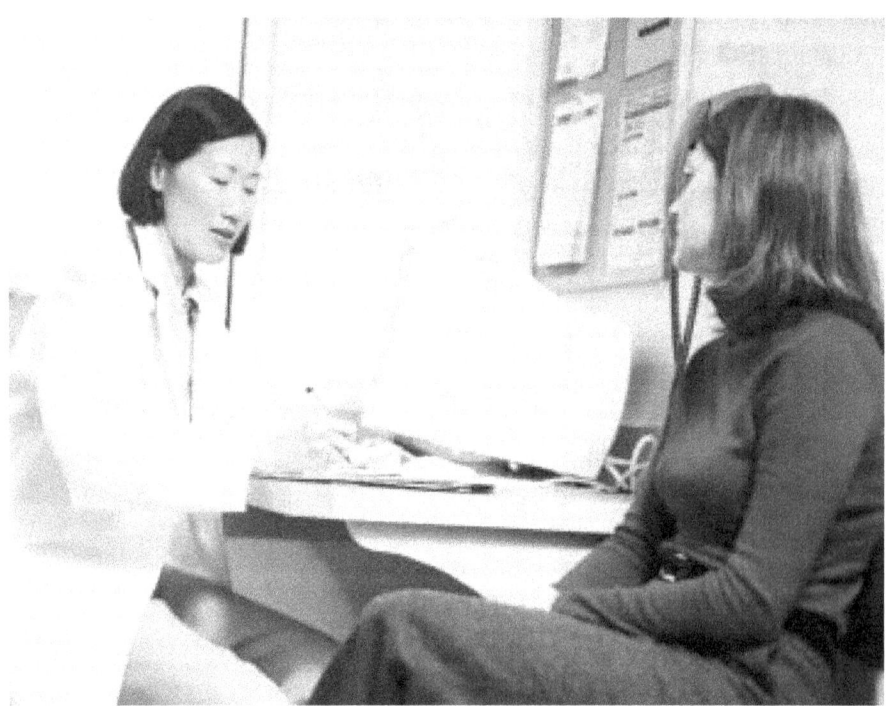

Decisions concerning eligibility for clinical trials are often complicated, requiring very specific medical information about the person's condition and previous treatment. For that reason, it is always preferable to have a health care professional familiar with the person's case make the initial contact with the clinical trials team. People making calls directly may have insufficient medical information, which may make decisions about eligibility difficult and frustrating—for both the person making the call and for the researcher taking the call.

Once contact with a clinical trial team is made, the clinical trial staff assists potential participants and their health care providers with information about potential clinical trials at the institution. Depending on the institution, a referral coordinator, protocol assistant, or nurse may accept telephone, mail, and e-mail inquiries from physicians, potential participants, and others about a clinical trial. Preliminary eligibility can be evaluated by phone, and appointments with the clinical trial team can be scheduled.

Both patients and health care providers can find specific trials through PDQ®, NCI's comprehensive cancer trial database. For more information on PDQ, see the following page.

Finding Information on Cancer and Clinical Trials

NCI Resources

NCI's Web site, *www.cancer.gov*, provides access to a wealth of information on clinical cancer care. The site contains information from PDQ®, including the latest information about cancer treatment, screening, prevention, genetics, supportive care, and complementary and alternative medicine, as well as a registry of cancer clinical trials. Clinical oncology specialists review current literature from more than 70 medical journals, evaluate its relevance, and synthesize it into clear summaries, which are then reviewed monthly and updated as needed based on new information. Most cancer information summaries appear in two versions: 1) a technical version for the health professional, and 2) a nontechnical version for patients, their families, and the public. Many of the summaries are also available in Spanish.

The NCI Web site also includes approximately 100 fact sheets on various cancer-related topics, information on ordering NCI publications, and educational features and news summaries concerning the latest results from cancer clinical trials.

NCI's clinical trials registry (PDQ) contains more than 1,800 ongoing clinical trials, including information about studies around the world. All clinical trials undergo review prior to inclusion. Although no single resource lists every cancer clinical trial being conducted in the United States and abroad, PDQ is the most comprehensive cancer clinical trials registry; it contains information about trials sponsored by NCI, the pharmaceutical industry, and some international groups. Users can narrow their search by multiple parameters, such as stage of disease, phase of trial, treatment modality, and geographic location. PDQ also contains an archival file of more than 11,000 clinical trials that are no longer accepting patients, including contact information for the principal investigators of trials that may not yet be published in the biomedical literature.

Accessing NCI's Clinical Trials and Cancer Information by Phone

NCI's Cancer Information Service—NCI's Cancer Information Service is a national information and education network for patients, the public, and health professionals. From regional offices covering the entire United States, Puerto Rico, and the U.S. Virgin Islands, trained staff provide the latest cancer information through a toll-free telephone service. Staff can respond to calls in either English or Spanish. With regional offices throughout the United States, CIS staff members may work with organizations and professionals to plan, implement, and evaluate culturally appropriate clinical trials education programs using the Clinical Trials Education Series.

> Access: The toll-free number is 1-800-4-CANCER (1-800-422-6237). For deaf and hard of hearing callers with TTY equipment, the number is 1-800-332-8615. Hours of operation are Monday through Friday, 9:00 a.m. to 4:30 p.m., local time. Callers also have the option of listening to recorded information about cancer 24 hours a day, 7 days a week.

NIH Web Site

It is important to note that there is no single resource that lists every cancer clinical trial being conducted in the United States and abroad. However, in 2000 the National Institutes of Health launched a new Web site, *www.clinicaltrials.gov*, that aims to be a complete listing of all U.S. Government- and industry-sponsored clinical trials, including cancer trials.

The site contains approximately 7,200 clinical trials, most of them Government-sponsored. However, additional trials from the pharmaceutical industry are being added.

Other Web Sites

The Internet includes a variety of clinical trial databases and matching services. The owners of these sites can be:

- Not-for-profit organizations, where the content providers may be volunteers and the site may be supported by an academic institution or foundation
- Companies that are heavily funded by investors who pharmaceutical companies pay every time a patient signs up for a clinical trial
- Something in between (e.g., a for-profit organization that gives some of its profits back to the cancer community)

Anyone interested in using any of these online services to find a clinical trial should ask a number of questions and evaluate the information before submitting personal information or calling an investigator from the service:

- Who owns/runs the site?
- Where does the financial backing come from?
- How does the service get paid? By matching people to trials? By clinical trial submission to the database? Other?
- Does anyone make money on this site? If so, then who?
- What is the source of clinical trial information?
- Does the site include all clinical trials? All Government-supported trials? All pharmaceutical trials?

Most people would like to have all of their treatment/prevention choices presented in an unbiased way before they make important health-related decisions. People may wish to look at the information from many of these sites and consider the source of the information before deciding what actions to take.

Guide To Finding Clinical Trial Resources

	What is it?	How do I access it?	What will it provide?
National Cancer Institute's PDQ	Database produced by NCI Registry of approximately 1,800 active cancer clinical trials	Go to *www.cancer.gov* Go to the clinical trials area and follow the search directions OR Call 1-800-4-CANCER	Summaries about clinical trials conducted by NCI-sponsored researchers, the pharmaceutical industry, and some international groups
National Library of Medicine	Database produced by NIH Registry now lists 4,000 primarily NIH-supported clinical studies on many conditions, and more will be added All trials on PDQ are listed in this database	Go to *www.clinicaltrials.gov* Can browse by disease or sponsor or insert key words	Summaries about clinical trials for a wide range of conditions—most of the trials listed are sponsored by NIH
Food and Drug Administration's Cancer Clinical Trials Directory	A list of sources prepared by FDA's Office of Special Health Issues Guides user to other Web locations for institutions that conduct or list cancer clinical trials	Go to *www.fda.gov/oashi/cancer/trials.html#table* Can browse by disease for different sources	Web addresses and telephone numbers Information listed on the Web sites in this directory varies widely
Local Cancer Center Web Sites	Locally produced Web sites that include listings for trials sponsored by NCI and some pharmaceutical companies Good supplementary resources for locating clinical trials; a cancer center may begin participating in an NCI-sponsored trial before the center's information is listed in CancerNet/PDQ	Different sites can be found through: • *www.cancer.gov* • Local institutions • Call 1-800-4-CANCER for a center near you Information on trials taking place at NCI's Clinical Center in Bethesda, Maryland is available at *http://ccr.nci.nih.gov* then select "clinical trials" Some centers may also have telephone information centers	Information that varies from center to center
Example of Pharmaceutical Resources/ Internet Clinical Trial Matching Sites	Pharmaceutical Research and Manufacturers of America (PhRMA) publishes a list of new cancer drugs in development CenterWatch's Clinical Trials Listing Service and EmergingMed.com's clinical trials matching service list many industry- and Government-sponsored trials	**PhRMA** Go to *http://www.phrma.org* Click on "New Medicines in Development" and search by disease. The drugs are listed by cancer type or call 202-835-3400. **CenterWatch** Go to *www.centerwatch.com* Click on "Trial Listings" and then "CenterWatch Trial Listings by Medical Areas" or call 617-856-5900. **EmergingMed.com** Go to *http://www.emergingmed.com*	Descriptions, sites, telephone numbers, and investigator names by State

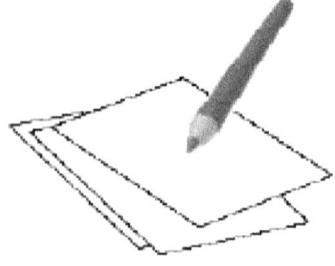

Exercises

Exercise 5.1

Involvement in Clinical Trials

If a doctor seems too busy to refer a person to a clinical trial, can the person make the calls directly?

_____

_____

_____

_____

Answer to Exercise 5.1

Decisions concerning eligibility for clinical trials
may be complicated, often requiring very specific medical
information on the person's condition.

- It is usually preferable to have the contact made by a doctor
  familiar with the case.
- Potential participants making direct calls may
  have insufficient information, which may make
  decisions about eligibility difficult.
- Depending on the institution, a member of the research team
  may accept telephone, mail, and e-mail inquiries from
  physicians, potential participants, and others
  about the clinical trial. In this case, preliminary eligibility can
  be evaluated by phone, and appointments with the
  clinical trial team can be scheduled.

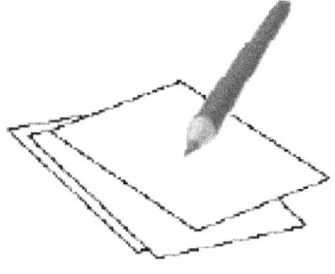

Exercise 5.2

Using PDQ to Locate Clinical Trials in Your Community

Choose two cancer diagnoses from the list below. Using *www.cancer.gov*, locate at least three clinical trials going on in your city or state.

When you have found at least three open trials, print out the patient versions and answer the question below. You can use NCI's PDQ or ask for printouts by calling 1-800-4-CANCER.

A. Someone diagnosed with stage II ovarian cancer who is looking for treatment options in your city and state

B. Someone diagnosed with stage IV colon cancer who needs options for supportive care

C. Someone diagnosed with stage III small cell lung cancer who needs options for treatment

D. Someone who is found to be at high risk for breast cancer who needs options for prevention

Question
What did you learn about clinical trials in your community or State?

_____

_____

_____

_____

Glossary

adverse effect: See *side effects*.

agent: In a cancer clinical trial, an agent is a substance that produces, or is capable of producing, an effect that fights cancer.

anthracycline: A member of a family of anticancer drugs that are also antibiotics.

bias: Human choices, beliefs, or any other factors besides those being studied that affect a clinical trial's results. Clinical trials use many methods to avoid bias because biased results may not be accurate.

biological therapy: Treatment to stimulate or restore the ability of the immune system to fight infection and disease. Also used to lessen side effects that may be caused by some cancer treatments. Also known as immunotherapy, biotherapy, or biological response modifier (BRM) therapy.

cancer: A term for diseases in which abnormal cells divide without control. Cancer cells can invade nearby tissues and can spread through the bloodstream and lymphatic system to other parts of the body.

cancer vaccine: A form of biological therapy which may help a person's immune system to recognize cancer cells. These vaccines may help the body reject tumors and prevent cancer from recurring.

chemoprevention: The use of drugs, vitamins, or other agents to try to reduce the risk of or delay the development or recurrence of cancer.

chemotherapy: Treatment with anticancer drugs.

clinical trial: A research study that tests how well new medical treatments or other interventions work in people. Each study is designed to test new methods of screening, prevention, diagnosis, or treatment of a disease.

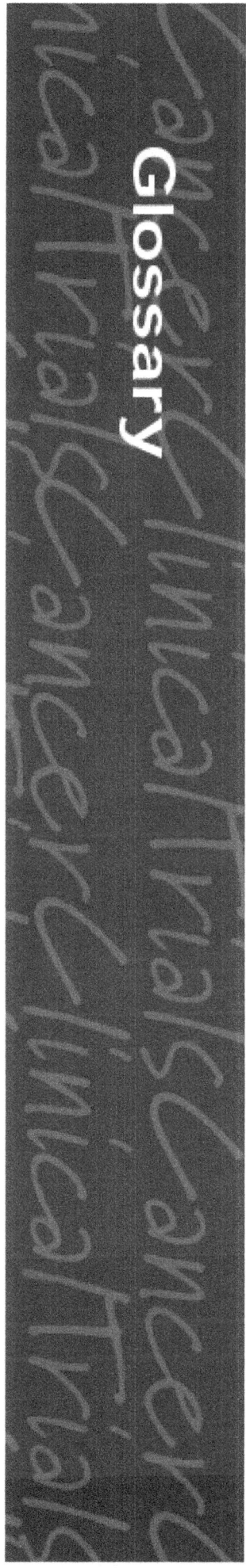

Community Clinical Oncology Program (CCOP): A program that links community physicians with NCI clinical research programs, enabling more people with cancer to participate in clinical trials in their own communities.

control group: In a randomized clinical trial, the group that receives standard treatment.

cooperative groups: Networks of institutions that jointly carry out large clinical trials following the same protocols.

data and safety monitoring board (DSMB): An independent committee whose membership includes, at minimum, a statistician and a clinical expert in the area being studied. Responsibilities of the DSMB are to: ensure that risks associated with participation are minimized to the extent possible, ensure the integrity of the data, and stop a trial either if safety concerns arise or as soon as its objectives have been met.

diagnostic trial: A research study that evaluates methods of detecting disease.

eligibility criteria: Participant eligibility criteria for clinical trials can range from general (age, sex, type of cancer) to specific (prior treatment, tumor characteristics, blood cell counts, organ function). Eligibility criteria may also vary with trial phase. In phase 1 and 2 trials, the criteria often focus on making sure that people who might be harmed because of abnormal organ function or other factors are not put at risk. Phase 2 and 3 trials often add criteria regarding disease type and stage, and number of prior treatments.

endpoint: What researchers measure to evaluate the results of a new treatment being tested in a clinical trial. Research teams establish the endpoints of a trial before it begins. Examples of endpoints include toxicity, tumor response, survival time, and quality of life.

Food and Drug Administration (FDA): An agency of the U.S. Department of Health and Human Services whose mission it is to promote and protect the public health: 1) by ensuring that medical products are proven safe and effective before they can be used by patients and 2) by monitoring products for continued safety after they are in use.

gene: The functional and physical unit of heredity passed from parent to offspring. Genes are pieces of DNA, and most genes contain the information for making a specific protein.

gene therapy: Treatment that alters a gene. In studies of gene therapy for cancer, researchers are trying to improve the body's natural ability to fight the disease or to make the cancer cells more sensitive to other kinds of therapy.

genetic: Inherited; having to do with information that is passed from parents to offspring through genes in sperm and egg cells.

genetic testing: Analyzing DNA to look for a genetic alteration that may indicate an increased risk for developing a specific disease or disorder.

genetics research: Research that focuses on how someone's genetic makeup can assist in the early detection, diagnosis, or treatment of cancer. Genetics research may be a part of screening or treatment trials.

investigational group: In a clinical trial, the group that receives the new agent being tested. See also *control group*.

imaging: Tests that produce pictures of areas inside the body.

immune system: The complex group of organs and cells that defends the body against infection or disease.

immunotherapy: See *biological therapy*.

informed consent: The process of providing all relevant information about the trial's purpose, risks, benefits, alternatives, and procedures to a potential participant, who then, consistent with his or her own interests and circumstances, makes an informed decision about whether to participate.

institutional review board (IRB): A board designed to oversee the research process in order to protect participant safety. Made up of researchers, ethicists, and lay people from the community, the board must review the trial protocols and the informed consent forms participants sign.

investigational new drug (IND): A drug that the Food and Drug Administration (FDA) allows to be used in clinical trials, but that the FDA has not yet approved for commercial marketing.

monoclonal antibodies: A form of biological therapy that may help the body's own immune system fight cancer by locating cancer cells and either killing them or delivering cancer-killing substances to them without harming normal cells.

oncology: The branch of medicine that deals with tumors, including study of their development, diagnosis, treatment, and prevention.

National Cancer Institute (NCI): Part of the National Institutes of Health of the United States Department of Health and Human Services, is the Federal Government's principal agency for cancer research. NCI conducts, coordinates, and funds cancer research, training, health information dissemination, and other programs with respect to the cause, diagnosis, prevention, and treatment of cancer. Access the NCI Web site at *www.cancer.gov*.

New Drug Application (NDA): The application filed with FDA by the trial sponsor once a trial has generated adequate data to support a certain indication for a drug (usually by finding that the drug is safe and superior to standard treatment in a definitive phase 3 trial).

Office for Human Research Protections (OHRP): This office safeguards participants in federally funded research and provides unity and leadership for many federal departments and agencies that carry out research involving human participants.

phase 1 trial: Small groups of people with cancer are treated with a certain dose of a new agent that has already been extensively studied in the laboratory. During the trial, the dose is usually increased group by group in order to find the highest dose that does not cause harmful side effects. This process determines a safe and appropriate dose to use in a phase 2 trial.

phase 2 trial: Phase 2 trials continue to test the safety of the new agent and begin to evaluate how well it works against a specific type of cancer. In these trials, the new agent is given to groups of people with one type of cancer or related cancers, using the dosage found to be safe in phase 1 trials.

phase 3 trial: Phase 3 studies are designed to answer research questions across the disease continuum. Phase 3 trials usually have hundreds to thousands of participants, in order to find out if there are true differences in the effectiveness of the treatment being tested.

phase 4 trial: Phase 4 trials are used to evaluate the long-term safety and effectiveness of a treatment. Less common than phase 1, 2, and 3 trials, phase 4 trials take place after the new treatment has been approved for standard use.

Physician Data Query (PDQ): PDQ is an online database developed and maintained by the National Cancer Institute. Designed to make the most current, credible, and accurate cancer information available to health professionals and the public, PDQ contains peer-reviewed summaries on cancer treatment, screening, prevention, genetics, and supportive care; a registry of cancer clinical trials from around the world; and directories of physicians, professionals who provide genetics services, and organizations that provide cancer care.

placebo: A treatment, often a drug, designed to look like the medicine being tested but that doesn't contain any active ingredient. Some people call a placebo a "sugar pill." Placebos are almost never used in cancer treatment trials.

preclinical testing: A process in which scientists test promising new anticancer agents in the laboratory and in animal models. This is done to find out whether agents have an anticancer effect and are safely tolerated in animals. Once a drug proves promising in the lab, the sponsor applies for FDA approval to test it in clinical trials involving people.

prevention trials: Trials involving healthy people who are at high risk for developing cancer. These trials try to answer specific questions about and evaluate the effectiveness of ways to reduce the risk of cancer.

principal investigator (PI): The person, usually a doctor, who is in charge of a clinical trial. The PI prepares a protocol for the trial.

protocol: A written plan that acts as a "recipe" for conducting a clinical trial. The protocol explains what a trial will do, how it will be carried out, and why each part of the trial is necessary.

quality of life: The overall enjoyment of life. Many clinical trials measure aspects of an individual's sense of well-being and ability to perform various tasks to assess the effects of cancer and its treatment on the quality of life.

radiation therapy: The use of high-energy radiation from x-rays, gamma rays, neutrons, and other sources to kill cancer cells and shrink tumors. Radiation may come from a machine outside the body (external-beam radiation therapy) or it may come from radioactive material placed in the body in the area near cancer cells (internal radiation therapy, implant radiation, or brachytherapy). Systemic radiation therapy uses a radioactive substance, such as a radiolabeled monoclonal antibody, that circulates throughout the body. Also called radiotherapy.

randomization: A method used to prevent bias in research. A computer generates treatment assignments, and participants have an equal chance to be assigned to one of two or more groups (e.g., the control group or the investigational group).

randomized clinical trial: A study in which the participants are assigned by chance to separate groups that compare different treatments; neither the researchers nor the participants can choose which group. Using chance to assign people to groups means that the groups will be similar and that the treatments they receive can be compared objectively. At the time of the trial, it is not known which treatment is best. It is the patient's choice to be in a randomized trial.

remission: A decrease in or disappearance of signs and symptoms of cancer. In partial remission, some, but not all, signs and symptoms of cancer have disappeared. In complete remission, all signs and symptoms of cancer have disappeared, although there still may be cancer in the body.

screening: Checking for disease when there are no symptoms.

screening trials: Clinical trials that focus on what tests can help find cancer in people before they have any cancer symptoms. The goal of early detection/screening trials is to discover new methods for finding cancer as early as possible. For many types of cancer, the ability to find and treat the disease at an early stage provides a better chance for survival.

side effects: Problems that occur when treatment affects healthy cells. Common side effects of cancer treatment are fatigue, nausea, vomiting, decreased blood cell counts, hair loss, and mouth sores.

stage: The extent of a cancer, especially whether the disease has spread from the original site to other parts of the body.

standard treatment: A currently accepted and widely used treatment for a certain type of cancer, based on the results of past research.

toxicity: Harmful side effects from an agent being tested.

treatment trials: Clinical trials conducted to examine new treatment approaches for people who have cancer and to determine the most effective treatments.

tumor: An abnormal mass of tissue that results from excessive cell division. Tumors perform no useful body function. They may be benign (not cancerous) or malignant (cancerous).

vaccine: A substance or group of substances meant to cause the immune system to respond to a tumor or to microorganisms, such as bacteria or viruses.

Notes

www.ingramcontent.com/pod-product-compliance
Lightning Source LLC
Chambersburg PA
CBHW081550170526
45166CB00009B/2647